INFECTION CONTROL

Edited by **Silpi Basak**

Infection Control
http://dx.doi.org/10.5772/56704
Edited by Silpi Basak

Contributors

Hiroshi Eguchi, Georgios Meletis, Silpi Basak, Monali Rajurkar, Ruchita Attal, Sanjay Mallick, Lul Raka

Published by InTech

Janeza Trdine 9, 51000 Rijeka, Croatia

Publishing Process Manager Oliver Kurelic
Technical Editor InTech DTP team
Cover InTech Design team

Additional hard copies can be obtained from orders@intechopen.com

Infection Control, Edited by Silpi Basak
p. cm.
ISBN 978-953-51-1145-0

For EU product safety concerns:
IN TECH d.o.o., Prolaz Marije Krucifikse Kozulić 3, 51000 Rijeka, Croatia, info@intechopen.com or visit our website at intechopen.com.

Meet the editor

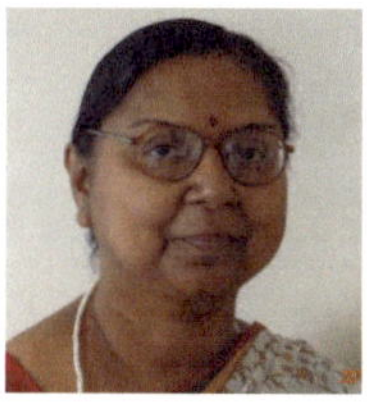

Dr. Silpi Basak has a vast experience in Infection Control practices in Health Care setup. Dr.S.Basak is working as Professor and Head of the Department of Microbiology, Jawaharlal Nehru Medical College, Wardha (M.S.) – 442004, India. She has been teaching Microbiology to M.B.B.S., B.D.S. and M.D. Microbiology students for 24 years. She has attended many State and National conferences and presented papers. She has conducted National Hands on Training on Polymerase Chain Reaction (PCR) in 2008 and 2009. She has 30 publications in National and International journals. She has also published 5 chapters in books. She is a reviewer in the Journal of Clinical Diagnostics and Research. Her field of research is Resistance to Antimicrobial drugs and Infection Control Practices.

Contents

Preface

Health Care associated infection (HAI) is an emerging problem worldwide. HAI causes increased morbidity and mortality and average length of stay of the patient in the hospital. HAI also imposes economic burden on the patient, health care set up and also State and National Health care system. Infection control in health care set up is a team work. It is the responsibility of all the persons associated with patient care.

I still remember how much I felt desperate, when I found that Pseudomonas aeruginosa and Candida albicans were isolated from Endotracheal aspirate of my mother who was admitted in OTICU and was having Ventilator Associated Pneumonia (VAP).

It has been estimated that 5 – 10 % of all hospital admission suffers from HAI even in developed countries. But 30% of HAI are preventable, if we follow the infection control practices properly especially hand hygiene while giving patient care. Hence, in this book importance has been given to Infection Control practices along with emerging trends of HAI.

Dr. Silpi Basak, M.B.B.S., M.D.
Department of Microbiology, Jawaharlal Nehru Medical College,
Sawangi (M) Wardha, India

Section 1

Facets of Infection Control Practices in Health Care Set Up

Chapter 1

Infection Control Practices in Health Care Set-Up

Silpi Basak, Monali N. Rajurkar, Sanjay K. Mallick and Ruchita O. Attal

Additional information is available at the end of the chapter

http://dx.doi.org/10.5772/55029

1. Introduction

"...... the very first requirement in a hospital is that it should do the sick no harm"

- Florence Nightingale

In India, Egypt, Palestine and Greece, the concept of hospital with hygienic practices was present as early as 500 BC. Later, hospitals became overcrowded as it were only meant for military personnel [1]. From 18th Century onwards new hospitals were established for civilians also. The transmission of infections in the hospital were also known to mankind since the sick were housed together for treatment. But no epidemiological data or surveillance system was available. But the enormity of the problem of Hospital Acquired Infections in pre-Lister era can be best understood by the writing of John Bell in 1801 who described the concept of "Hospital Gangrene" [2]. Lord Joseph Lister first used carbolic acid as an antiseptic in 1865 and published his work in 1867 which started the antiseptic era and he has been remembered as "Father of Antiseptic Surgery".

Louis Pasture in his celebrated lecture to Academic de Medicine on 30th April, 1873 said, "If I had the honour of being a surgeon.... not only would I use absolutely clean instruments (free from germs) but after cleaning my hands with great care would only use sponges previously raised to a heat of 130-150^0 F. I would still have to fear germs suspended in air and surrounding of the patient" [2].

So with progressive awareness in later part of 16th century, regarding the transmission of infection among hospitalized patients continued to be a great concern for everyone related to hospitals but still hospital acquired infections remain a problem worldwide even today. World

Health Organisation (WHO) conducted a survey and the results of the survey in 1988 reported that "Hospital Acquired Infection is a considerable problem even in hospitals in which means and interests in control of Hospital Acquired Infections exist" [2].

British Medical Council established Hospital Infection Control Programme in 1941 and a part time post of "Control Of Infection Officer" was created, which was renamed as "Infection Control Doctor" in 1988. The first full time "Infection Control Nurse" was appointed in 1959 [1]. National Nosocomial Infections Surveillance (NNIS) system of the Centre for Disease Control and Preventions (CDC) was developed in early 1970s to monitor the incidence of Hospital Acquired Infection, the risk factors and causative organisms [3].

The term nosocomial infection is derived from nosus means disease and komeion means to take care of and has been used for many years. The hospital acquired or nosocomial infections have been defined as infections that occur to patients during hospitalization but are neither present nor incubating during admission to the hospital. In simple words, any infections acquired in a hospital which was not present or in its incubation period during admission to the hospital are called nosocomial infections.

In the past, nosocomial infections or Hospital Acquired Infections were restricted only to the hospitals, but in recent years, spectrum of health care and interactions of different types of healthcare facilities including hospital, long term care, rehabilitation or ambulatory care facilities have been expanded and nosocomial infections have broadened its horizon. Hence, the term Healthcare Associated Infection (HAI) is a more appropriate term. The Centers for Disease Control and Prevention (CDC) defines HAIs as infections that patients acquire during the course of receiving treatment for other conditions or that Healthcare workers (HCWs) acquire while performing their duties within a healthcare setting [4]. The bacterial HAIs are usually observed, 48 hours after admission to healthcare setup, because for most of the routinely isolated bacteria the incubation period is 48 hours. But each infection must be assessed individually as the incubation period varies with the type of pathogen, dose of inoculum and patient's immune status. Some HAIs may be observed even after discharge of the patient especially, Hepatitis B virus (HBV), Hepatitis C virus (HCV), Human immune deficiency virus (HIV) etc. Even CDC has changed the name of section of Hospital Infections Programme to the Division of Healthcare Quality Promotion [5]. The National Health care safety network (NHSN) of CDC defines HAI as a localized or systemic condition that results from presence of infectious agent or its toxin and that was not present or incubating at the time of admission to the Hospital / Health care facility [6].

2. HAI is on the rise

In last century mankind has experienced tremendous advancement in Medical field in understanding the causes and thereby improvement in diagnostic and therapeutic approach of any disease. Similarly, progress in engineering field has changed the look of Health care system. But with all these advancements also, HAIs are on the rise mainly because of -

i. Increase in immunocompromised patients

ii. Interward and interhospital or interhealth care facility transfer

iii. Emergence of antibiotic resistant bacteria prevalent in Health care facilities

iv. Increased work load – Staff pressure, Lack of facilities, Lack of concern ???

The last one is most dangerous. Though scenario is slightly better in developed world the picture is grim in other developing countries. According to WHO report 2002 [7] worldwide more than 1.4 million people suffer from HAI. Actually HAI vary from 5-25% in developed countries, whereas data from developing country is not available as it is not reported properly. It may be >40% in Asia, Africa and South America [8]. Klevens et al, 2007 had reported that HAIs killed 99,000 patients in American hospital [9] and 37,000 deaths in Europe [10]. In US, 5-10% of all hospitalized patients can get HAI. In India data are sparse, Mukherjee V had reported in 2001 that HAI occurred in 30-35% of all hospital admissions in India [11]. Childs D reported that HAIs kill more patients every year than do AIDS, breast cancer and automobile accidents together worldwide [12]. HAIs are the 8th most common cause of death in US. The mortality rate range from 12-80% in ICUs of developed countries [13].

Impact of HAI

The major impact of HAI are outcome of disease is adversely affected. HAI is the major cause of: i) increased morbidity and mortality, ii) increased average length of stay (ALS) of patients in the Health Care set up, iii) increased diagnostic and therapeutic interventions and iv) increased cost of Health Care. HAI adds financial burden to patients, health care organization, State and also National Health Care system. HAI also have negative impact on effectiveness and productivities of Health Care organization. In case of HAI, patients are not protected by Health insurance and the health care organization comes under consumer protection act.

The triad of infectious diseases as described in textbooks are i). the affected host ii). an infectious agent and iii). the environment, both animate and inanimate [14]. HAIs also follow the same triad as the affected host may be the patients, health care workers(HCW), patient's relatives, the infectious agent may be Methicillin Resistant Staphylococcus aureus(MRSA), Vancomycin Resistant Enterococci(VRE), Pseudomonas aeruginosa, other Gram negative bacteria or simply Candida, Aspergillus or viral e.g. Cytomegalovirus, HBV, HIV etc and most important the hospital environment.

Hence, the epidemiological triad of HAI are –

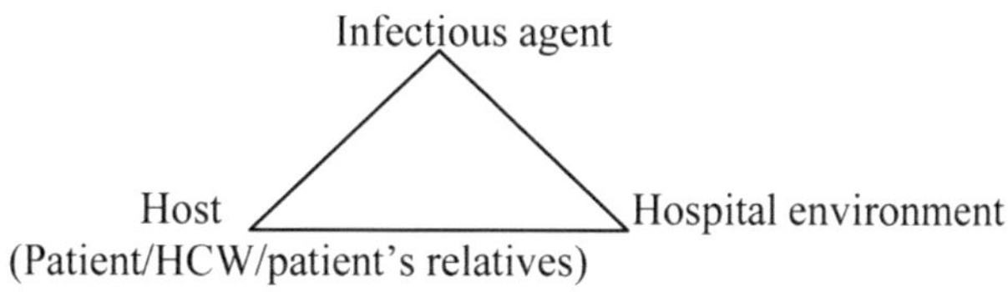

2.1. The high risk areas for HAI

Nurseries, Intensive care units (ICUs), Operation theatres (OTs) and Post operative wards, Labour room, Dialysis unit, Organ transplant unit, Oncology wards, Burn units, High Dependency units (HDU) etc are mainly high risk areas for HAI.

2.2. Host factors responsible for HAI

i. Repeated hospital admissions

ii. Increased number of patients receiving intensive care or long term care facilities

iii. Extremes of age i.e. in elderly patients the immunity is waning and in newborn the immune system is immature

iv. Increased survival of low birth weight or premature babies treated in NICUs

v. Increased incidence of road accidents leading to head injury, spinal cord injury in trauma ICUs

vi. Patients with diabetes, malnutrition

vii. Patients with HIV / AIDS etc

2.3. Source of HAI

HAIs acquired by a patient may be endogenous (autogenous) and exogenous. Endogenous infections are caused by patient's own flora or by carrier state, whereas exogenous infections result from transmission of organisms from various sources via different routes [15]. Exogenous sources may be other patients with infectious diseases. HCWs carrying MRSA, Multidrug resistant (MDR) Gram negative organisms on hands or dresses, contaminated disinfectant solutions, environmental surfaces especially frequently – touched surfaces e.g. bed rails, furnitures, door latches, toilet seats, telephones etc and even floor, window panes, air conditioners, renovation work, inefficient sterilization of equipment and devices. Moreover, medications or devices, necessary to cure patient's primary medical condition can also predispose to HAI. The important ones are -

i. Overuse or injudicious use of antimicrobials

ii. Indwelling medical devices such as urinary catheters, endotracheal tubes, ventilators, artificial heart valves, joint prosthesis etc which break the body's natural barrier to infection, which can also lead to biofilm formation and form a nidus for chronic persistent infection.

iii. Improper maintenance of operation theatres and ICUs etc

2.4. The mode of transmission of HAI may be

Contact (direct or indirect), droplet, airborne, common vehicle (food, water, medical devices, blood or blood products etc) and vector borne (mosquitos, flies, rats etc)

http://dx.doi.org/10.5772/55029

Contact transmission : The organisms which are transmitted by contact are MRSA, VRE etc.

Direct contact transmission occurs direct body surface to body surface contact and commonly occurs to HCW [16], while giving patient care. Indirect contact transmission occurs with contaminated inanimate objects e.g. needles, dressings, contaminated hands of HCW, endoscopes etc.

Droplets are generated while coughing, sneezing, talking or performing suctioning, bronchoscopy etc. The droplets (large particles >5μm in size) transmitted from infected person through air (short distance ≤ 3 feet) and deposited on host's conjunctiva, nasal mucosa or mouth. But the droplets are not suspended in air [15].

Airborne transmission occurs by airborne droplet nuclei (small particle ≤ 5 μm in size) which are evaporated droplets containing the microorganisms that remain suspended in air for few hours or days. Mycobacterium tuberculosis, Varicella, Rubella, Influenza viruses etc can be transmitted by droplet nuclei [15].

2.5. Infecting agents

The organisms causing HAI are mostly antibiotic resistant, which adds to the increased morbidity and mortality of patients.

- Antibiotic resistant pathogens associated with HAI are –
- Major Gram positive pathogens
- Vancomycin Resistant Enterococci (VRE)
- Methicillin Resistant Staphylococcus aureus (MRSA)
- Methicillin Resistant Coagulase negative Staphylococci (MRCONS)
- Vancomycin Resistant Staphylococcus aureus (VRSA)
- Vancomycin Intermediate Staphylococcus aureus (VISA)
- Penicillin Resistant Pneumococci
- Major Gram negative pathogens :

Specially Extended spectrum β – lactamase (ESBL producing) or multi / Extreme drug Resistant Gram negative bacteria e.g.

- Pseudomonas aeruginosa
- Enterobacteriaceae : Klebsiella pneumoniae, E.coli, Citrobacter sp., Enterobacter sp. etc.
- Acinetobacter baumani
- Penicillinase producing Neisseria gonorrhoeae (PPNG)
- Burkholderia species, Stenotrophomonas maltophila and amongst fungi especially Fluconazole resistant Candida species are also becoming important agents causing HAI specially in ICU patients [17].

The terms Multidrug resistance and Extreme drug resistance in Gram negative bacteria was introduced by Falagas in 2011 [18]. Multidrug resistance (MDR) is indicated by non-susceptibility to one or more antibiotics belonging to 3 or more antibiotic classes, whereas Extreme drug resistance (XDR) is indicated by resistance to all available antibiotics.

In 2009, Peterson et al used the acronym ESCAPE for MDR organism causing HAI [19].

E : Enterococcus faecium/E.faecalis

S : Staphylococcus aureus

C : Clostridium difficile

A : Acinetobacter baumani

P : Pseudomonas aeruginosa

E : Enterobacteriaceae

10-12 % of all HAIs are caused by Enterococci which is the 3rd most common cause of blood stream infection in hospitalized patients. Vancomycin resistant Enterococci (VRE) was first isolated in vitro in 1969 and was described clinically in 1988. The main mechanism is alteration of cell wall precursors. Several resistant genotypes have been detected, of which vanA and vanB are most clinically significant. Vancomycin resistance is transferable to Staphylococcus aureus in vitro. As a life saving measure, treatment option with MDRO is very selective. MRSA strains can be treated by Vancomycin and Linezolid, VRE can be treated by Linezolid; ESBL producers can be treated by β – lactamase inhibitors; both ESBL and AmpC producers can be treated by Carbapenems. But Carbapenem resistant organisms can be treated by Colistin.

Recent studies in India have reported ESBL in 70 – 90% of Enterobacteriaceae, 29% Pseudomonas aeruginosa and 26% of Acinetobacter spp. which is a serious problem [20]. Recently from our hospital prevalence of AmpC β – lactamase and metallobetalactamase (MBL) producing P.aeruginosa strains have been reported as 19.3% in 2009 and 11.4% in 2010 respectively [21], [22].

3. HAI : Types by site

i. Unary tract infections (UTI) – UTI are mostly catheter associated which are called CA – UTI. CA – UTI are the second most common cause of health care associated Blood stream infections. As per National Health care Safety Network [23], CA – UTIs are defined as the patient having indwelling urinary catheter or 48 hours before onset of UTI. No time period is fixed that the patient must be having catheter to call UTI as CA – UTIs. Richards et al have reported in 1999 that 95% of UTIs in hospitals are CA – UTI. In CA – UTI not only bacteruria occurs but Candida albicans and Candida non-albicans species are also isolated and so a new term microburia has been introduced [24].

ii. Hospital acquired pneumonia (HAP) – is the second most common hospital acquired infection and accounts for 15% of HAIs [25]. Highest morbidity and mortality amongst all types of HAIs occur in HAP [26] and roughly the mortality range from 24 to 76 % in different health care settings [27]. Ventilator associated pneumonia (VAP) is the commonest cause of HAP which occurs after 48 hours of initiating mechanical ventilation [25], [28]. VAP occurs 25% of all ICU infections and caused by multidrug resistant bacteria e.g. Pseudomonas aeruginosa, Acinetobacter baummani or Carbepenemase producing Enterobacteriaceae, MRSA, VRE etc. Burkholderia sp. and Stenotrophomonas maltophila both have a tendancy to colonize respiratory tract rather than to cause invasive disease and are mostly resistant to Carbapenems, because of production of metallobetalactamase(MBL). The high mortality, prolonged ICU stay and excessive cost associated with VAP is a real challenge to medical fraternity.

iii. Surgical site infections (SSI) – SSIs are the most common nosocomial infection. SSIs are caused by MRSA, VRSA, VISA, VRE, Pseudomonas aeruginosa, Acinetobacter baumani, ESBL and AmpC β – lactamase producing E.coli, Klebsiella, Proteus etc and also by MBL and Klebsiella pneumoniae carbapenemase (KPC) producing Gram negative bacilli. SSIs occur when microorganisms gain access to areas of the body, exposed during surgical procedures and then multiply in the tissues. Mangram et al have defined SSIs which manifests within 30 days of a surgical procedure or within one year if the implant is left in place during the operative procedure and affect either the incision or deep tissue at the site of operation [29]. The intraoperative factors as proper skin preparation, following sterile techniques, traffic in the operating room contribute more to SSIs compared to patient related factors e.g. diabetes mellitus, pre existing colonization with MRSA etc [30]. SSIs are most commonly reported from surgical ward and CDC in US requires 16 wound and patient characteristics to define SSIs [31]. Though SSIs are preventable, about one fifth (approx. 22%) of all health care associated infections are due to SSIs (CDC report). Kirkland et al reported that 60% of patients with SSIs are ICU patients, average length of stay in hospital is >5 days and 5 times more likely to be readmitted in hospitals [32]. Hence, rates of SSIs are increasingly considered as a performance indicator for quality of health care provided.

iv. Catheter Related Blood Stream Infections (CR – BSIs) – These accounts for 50% of all ICU related bacteremias. CR – BSIs specially central line associated blood stream infections (CLABSIs) in ICU have been reported from USA as 1.8 to 5.2 per 1000 CVC catheter days where as studies from 8 developing countries reported the incidence as 12.5/1000 catheter days [33]. CR – BSIs are actually defined as bacteriaemia or fungiaemia in a patient who has an intravascular devise and a positive result of blood culture from peripheral vein, clinical manifestations and no other apparent source for BSI. The causative agents are Staphylococcus aureus even MRSA, Coagulase negative Staphylococci (CONS), Enterococcus species even VRE, Candida species, Pseudomonas aeruginosa, ESBL and Carbapenemase producing E.coli and Klebsiella, Burkholderia species etc. Candida species are known to cause CRBSIs in Neonatal ICU (NICU). Traditionally, Amphotericin B and Fluconazole are the only treatment options for invasive fungal disease in the neonate. Though C.albicans is mostly sensitive to Fluconazole, but Fluconazole resistant Candida species and toxicity with

Amphotericin B has made antifungal treatment more difficult for neonates. The new azole drug Voriconazole is used for invasive aspergillosis but this drug has not been studied in neonates and possibility of its effect on developing retina which is observed in adults and older children cannot be ruled out [34].

3.1. Scenario in our hospital, in last 5 years

Our hospital is a tertiary care hospital in a rural set up. Though actual incidence of HAI is difficult to calculate, mostly because of improper reporting system, in last 5 years, there is definitely an increase in isolation of Multiple drug resistant organisms (MDRO) from different clinical specimens.

In a study conducted from September 2007 to June 2008, out of 366 Staphylococcus aureus strains studied 189 (51.6%) strains were MRSA. Because of changing patterns of antibiotic resistance and emergence of MRSA, renewed interest in macrolides lincosamides and Streptogramin$_B$ (MLS_B) have been developed. Clindamycin, a semisynthetic derivative of Lincosamides has excellent tissue penetration (except in central nervous system), rapid oral absorption and no dose adjustment is required in renal insufficiency and it is one of the most efficient antibiotics in treating skin and soft tissue infections including osteomyelitis. Though the chemical structure of macrolide, lincosamides and streptogramin$_B$ are very different, their mechanism of action is identical i.e. to block protein synthesis by inhibiting peptidyl transferase. Bacteria develop cross resistance due to overlapping binding sites in 23 SrRNA. Three types of MLS_B resistance are observed -

i. Constitutive MLSB (cMLSB)

ii. Inducible MLSB (iMLSB) and

iii. MSB phenotype

For detection of $iMLS_B$ phenotype, D – zone test as per National Committee for Clinical Laboratory Standards (NCCLS) guideline 2004 is done [34]. In our study, out of 366 Staphylococcus aureus strains $iMLS_B$ (18.6%), $cMLS_B$ (3.8%) and MS_B(0.8%) phenotypes were detected respectively [35].

In another study, out of 280 Staphylococcus aureus strains 51.8% strains were MRSA. Out of these MRSA strains 61.4% were isolated from pus and wound swab and 13.8% MRSA strains were isolated from different ICUs (Medicine ICU, Neonatal ICU, Pediatric ICU, OT – ICU etc). 35.2% MRSA strains were $iMLS_B$ phenotype [36]. The MRSA strains were detected by Cetoxitin (30μg) disc diffusion test as per Clinical and Laboratory standards Institute guidelines [37]. These MRSA strains were further confirmed by doing PCR to detect mec A gene for MRSA and fem A gene for Staphylococcus aureus [38]. The increasing incidence of MRSA strains in our hospital could be compared with our study done in 1997 and at that time only 30.6% MRSA strains were isolated [39].

Presently, MDROs isolated from health care set up are mostly caused by different Gram negative organisms, which produce newer β – lactamases like ESBL, AmpC β – lactamases and metallobetalactamases(MBL).

http://dx.doi.org/10.5772/55029

From 2008 to 2010, out of total 250 Pseudomonas aeruginosa strains studied 40%, 42% and 11.2% were ESBL, AmpC β – lactamases and MBL producers respectively [40]. Amongst these ESBL and AmpC β – lactamase producers 27.2% P.aeruginosa strains produced both ESBL as well as AmpC β – lactamases. ESBL producing strains were detected by Combined disc method [41] and ESBL E - test strips [42]. AmpC β – lactamase was detected by Double disc synergy test and Disk potentiation test using 3 – aminophenyl boronic acid [43]. Metallobetalactamase (MBL) were detected by Imipenem – EDTA Double disc synergy test [44], Disk potentiation test [45] and were further confirmed by MBL E – test (AB bioMerieux) [46].

From different ICUs 59.4%MRSA strains were isolated and amongst Gram negative MDROs 21.5% only ESBL producers, 9.6% were only AmpC β – lactamase producers, 13.3% were both ESBL and AmpC β – lactamase producers and 15.6% strains were MBL producers [47]. 90.5% MBL producing strains were resistant to all 08 antibiotics used as per CLSI guidelines [37] and all 100% MBL producers were sensitive to Colistin [47].

In one of our study, 56 E.coli strains were isolated from different ICUs (Fig.1). 26(46.4%) strains isolated from different ICUs, produced both ESBL and AmpC β – lactamases(Fig.2). Maximum MBL producing E.coli strains 4 (7.8%) were isolated from Medicine ICU and High Dependency Unit(HDU). Only 01 E.coli strain was isolated from patient of HDU which produced all 3 types of β – lactamases i.e. ESBL, MBL and AmpC β – lactamases. The unpaired t test was performed with MBL producing and non – MBL producing E.coli stains isolated from MICU and HDU, NICU, PICU and OT – ICU and the probability of the result assuming null hypothesis was 0.043 and hence was significant.

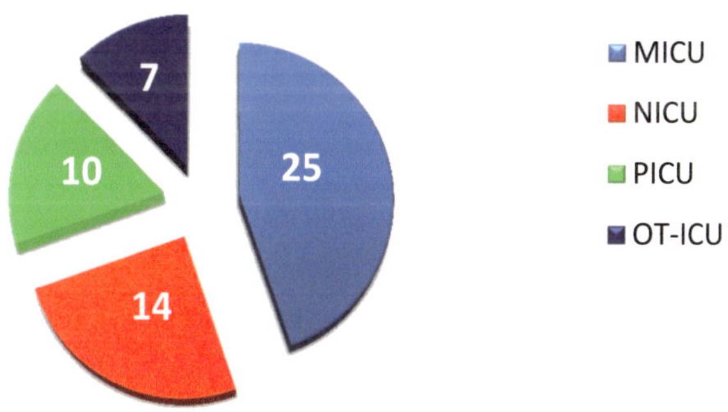

Figure 1. Isolation of *E.coli* strains from different ICUs (n = 56)

4. Infection control programme: Need of the hour

Every country develops a National Infection Control Programme to reduce the risk of Health Care Associated Infections (HAI) and thereby to achieve the national health care objectives with the help of a National Expert Committee. Each health care facility is required to develop an infection control programme to chalk out the annual work plan for monitoring and

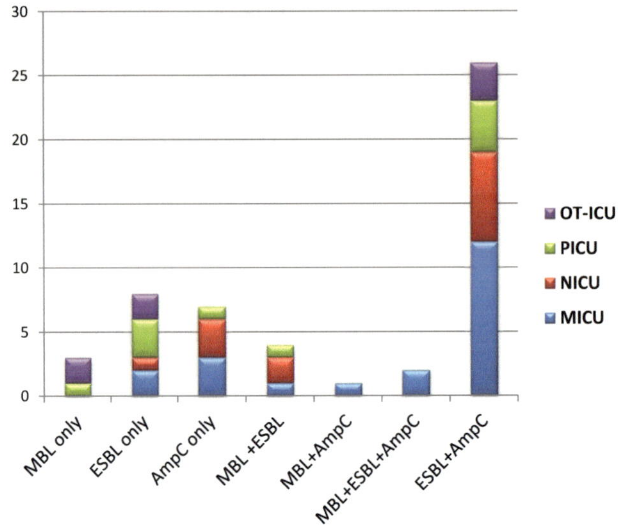

Figure 2. Isolation of ESBL, AmpC & MBL producing E.coli strains from different ICUs (n = 56)

surveillance of HAI, for educating, training health care workers (HCWs) in infection control practices, for controlling out breaks to ensure good health care to patients and prevention of infections for patients and staffs.

4.1. Hospital Infection Control Committee (HICC)

To have need based Infection Control Programme every Health Care facility should form a Hospital Infection Control Committee (HICC) which provides a forum for multidisciplinary input and cooperation and information sharing and include administrators, Clinical Microbiologists, Pharmacologists, HCWs specially ICU and OT incharges, housekeeping, maintenance staffs etc.

4.1.1. HICC must have

- A chairperson from administrators
- Infection Control Practitioner / Officer
- Infection Control Nurse

HICC should meet regularly in every months but not less than 3 times a year.

4.2. Infection control team

Infection Control Team is responsible for day to day activities of HICC in a health care facilities. It usually should have Infection Control Practitioner and other members who give scientific and technical support to carry out surveillance programme and to implement infection control policies, to manage critical incidents, to conduct training activities and to review the impact of training amongst Health Care Workers (HCWs).

4.3. Infection control manual

Every Health care facilities should have their own Infection Control Manual which is usually prepared by Infection Control Team and approved by HICC and updated. The manual should always be accessible to Health Care Workers (HCWs).

4.4. Infection Control Practices : are grouped into 2 catagories [48] –

i. Standard precautions – i.e. basic infection control precautions

ii. Additional precautions – i.e. transmission based precautions

Standard Precautions include basic infection control practices which must be applied to all patients at all times without taking consideration of diagnosis or infection status. Standard precautions are essential to provide a high level of protection to patients, HCWs and visitors (relatives of patients).

4.4.1. Standard precautions include

- Hand hygiene
- Use of personal protective equipments (PPE)
- Precaution of needle stick / sharp injuries
- Proper handling of patient care equipments
- Environmental cleaning and spills management
- Biomedical waste management

4.4.2. Hand hygiene

Hand hygiene is the most important simplest practice to reduce the transmission of HAI, which has been described in early 19th century by Ignaz Semmelweiss, a 2nd year medical student that puerperal sepsis was mainly transmitted by the contaminated hands of clinicians who conducted delivery just after performing autopsy without washing their hands [49], [50]. Semmelweiss also proved in 1847 that incidence of puerperal sepsis, fever and maternal mortality due to puerperal sepsis could be greatly reduced by washing hands.

In 2005, WHO introduced first Global safety challenge 'Clean care is Safer care' for patient safety [51]. In 2006, guidelines on Hand Hygiene in Health care were published. The first Global hand washing day was observed on 15th October 2008. In April 2009, 3.6 million HCWs worldwide, registered themselves to comply with WHO's global challenge on Hand Hygiene. On 5th May 2009, WHO launched guidelines on Hand Hygiene and the theme was 'Save lives : Clean Your Hands' [52], [53]. There may be resident flora and transient flora which can colonize the hands of HCW. The transient flora colonizes the superficial layer of skin and are removed by hand hygiene. The pathogens like MRSA, VRE, Multidrug resistant Gram negative bacilli, Candida species causing HAI colonize hands of HCW during patient care simply while taking blood pressure or taking temperature etc. or from environment like the uniform, patient's locker, bed rail, bed linens, furnitures etc. The organisms like Staphylococcus aureus, MRSA, VRE can survive for months on inanimate objects.

Hand hygiene includes washing hands with soap and water, antimicrobial soap, antiseptic agents, alcohol – based hand rub or surgical hand scrub. Hepatitis C virus (HCV), Rhinoviruses, Adenoviruses and Rotavirus nucleic acid can be found on hands of HCW [52].

If hands of HCWs are visibly dirty or contaminated with proteinaceous material, blood or other body fluids of patients, the hands are to be washed with soap and water. An alcohol based hand rub must be used by HCWs when hands are not visibly soiled such as before having any direct contact with patients including taking pulse or blood pressure or lifting a patient, before donning sterile gloves and also after removing gloves, after contact with inanimate objects in patient's immediate environment or if moving from a contaminated body site to a clean body site of the patient etc.

The maximum incidence of hand contaminations are reported from critical care areas. Hence, to prevent cross transmission, motivation, training, availability of alcohol based hand rubs and repeated reminders are required for HCWs. In most Health care set up, actually following the hand hygiene practice is below 40% where it is indicated [54]. The most important cause for poor hand hygiene compliance is lack of knowledge of guidelines of protocols on hand hygiene, lack of institution priority, lack of role model among the colleagues or superiors (specially clinicians), lack of HCWs etc [55].

The HCWs are to be specifically explained that wearing gloves does not replace hand hygiene and contamination may occur while removing the gloves. Actually, hand hygiene should be a habit of HCW while giving patient care.

Selection of hand hygiene products and its easy availability is one the most important step to promote hand hygiene practices during patient care. The new CDC guidelines does not suggest any specific spectrum for a hand hygiene agent and any health care set up can select an agent depending on cost spectrum and the common causative organisms of HAI [56]. Hand hygiene agent used for post contamination must be bactericidal, fungicidal (yeast), virucidal. The agent having activity against unenveloped viruses should be used in peadiatrics (rotavirus) or in oncology units (parvovirus) etc. The agent with mycobactericidal activity should be used in tuberculosis and chest wards, fungicidal activity (moulds) in organ transplant units or AIDS patients are to be considered. Preoperative hand hygiene agent should at least contain bactericidal and fungicidal (yeasts) to reduce the risk of SSIs. Any hand hygiene agent should not cause skin irritation and should dry on its own. WHO advocates to follow formula for resource poor settings [57].

Formulation I contains ethanol 80% v/v, glycerol 1.45% v/v and hydrogen peroxide 0.125% v/v.

Formulation II contains isopropyl alcohol 75% v/v, glycerol 1.45% v/v and hydrogen peroxide 0.125% v/v.

http://dx.doi.org/10.5772/55029

4.4.3. Personal Protective Equipment (PPE)

PPE includes gloves, protective eye wear (goggles), masks, cap, apron, gown, shoe covers etc. PPE should be used when there is a chance to have contact with patient's blood, body fluids, excretion or secretion while giving patient care by – HCWs, support staffs including attendants, sweeper, laundry staffs, laboratory staffs and family members. Masks alongwith goggles or a face shield may be used for complete protection of the face [58]. PPE should be chosen according to the risk of exposure and always where contact with blood and body fluid may occur. HCWs may be well trained when and how to use PPE and should be explained properly that use of PPE does not replace hand hygiene. Disposable PPEs e.g. gloves, masks, protective eyewear, gowns should never be reused. PPEs should always be changed between patients. All HCWs should follow hand hygiene after removal of PPE. Single use PPE must be discarded or reusable PPE may be put in a bin to send it to laundry and then for sterilization.

Respiratory protection : To prevent inhalation of microorganism the respirator with N-95 or higher filtration can be used. These are recommended if exposure to patients with tuberculosis, SARS CO-V, influenza, Swine flu etc occurs or suspected.

In the current CDC guidelines regarding isolation precaution Respiratory Hygiene / Cough Etiquette are recommended for HCWs, patients and their relatives. Spatially separation (>3 foot) should be followed in persons with respiratory infection in common waiting areas of health care set up. To avoid inhalation of droplet nuclei, droplet precautions e.g. wearing mask are to be implemented for HCWs. Masks should never be confused with particulate respirators which are used to prevent inhalation of small particles contaminated with infectious agent.

4.4.4. Safe injection practices

The recommendations include :

- Always sterile, single use disposable needle and syringe for each injection is to be used.
- CDC recommends single dose vials instead of multiple dose vials, when used for multiple patients. Multidose vials are always discouraged, because HCWs commonly contaminate the vials.
- The intravenous fluid infusion sets are to be used for one patient only and discarded after use.

4.4.5. Infection control practices for lumbar puncture procedure [59]

The health Care Infection Control Practices Advisory Committee (HICPAC) in 2005 recommended that the HCW placing a catheter or injecting material into the spinal or epidural space must use a facemasks to prevent droplet transmission of oropharyngeal flora.

4.4.6. Patient care equipment

To prevent patient to patient transmission, instruments must be cleaned and sterilized. All patient care equipment soiled with blood, body fluids, secretions or excretions must be handled with care to prevent exposure to skin and mucous membranes, clothing and environment. All reusable equipments are to be cleaned and sterilized before using for another patient.

4.4.6.1 .High level disinfection (HLD), Intermediate level disinfection (ILD) and Low level disinfection (LLD) [60].

High level disinfection (HLD) is a process that kills all microorganisms except large numbers of bacterial spores. The Food and Drug Administration definition of HLD is a sterilant used for a shorter contact time to achieve 10^6 log kill of an Mycobacterium sp. HLD chemicals can also be used for sterilization only with extended exposure time. The examples are glutaraldehyde 2%, Hydrogen peroxide 7.5%, Hydrogen peroxide and peracetic acid 1% / 0.8%, Hypochlorite and hypochlorus acid i.e. 650-675 ppm and 400-450 ppm respectively etc. HLD can be used for heat – sensitive semi critical patient care equipments e.g. Gastrointestinal endoscopes, bronchoscopes etc.

Intermediate level disinfection (ILD) – ILD is defined as a disinfection procedure that is cidal for Mycobacteria, vegetative bacteria, most viruses and fungi but does not kill bacterial spores. Tuberculocide germicide does not prevent transmission of tuberculosis in health care set – ups. The term tuberculocide is used to denote germicidal potency of disinfectant. The examples of ILD are hypochlorite, alcohols, phenols etc. ILDs are mainly used for soiled noncritical patient care items or surfaces contaminated with visible blood/ body fluids/sputum/faeces/Mycobacteria.

Low level disinfection (LLD) is a process that kills most vegetative bacteria, some fungi and some viruses (lipophilic viruses) etc in ≤ 10 minutes. LLD includes some chlorine based products, phenolics and quaternary ammonium compounds or 70-90% alcohol. LLD is used for non critical patients care items.

4.4.6.2. Critical, semicritical & non critical devices

The definition of HLD, ILD and LLD correlates well with Spaulding's classification of devices [61]. The Equipment/device is defined as **Critical** if the medical device enter into a normally sterile tissue or vasculature and for reprocessing sterilization is required. The examples are cardiac catheter, needle, surgical instruments, implants etc.

The medical devices are called **Semicritical** if the device can come in contact with mucous membrane or non intact skin. For reprocessing, sterilization is desirable but HLD is acceptable. The examples are respiratory therapy equipment, some endoscopes etc.

The **Noncritical** devices can be defined as devices that come in contact with intact skin, e.g. Blood pressure cuff, Stethoscopes etc and for reprocessing ILD / LLD can be used.

4.4.6.3. Environmental surfaces

In 1991, CDC has proposed an additional category as 'Environmental surfaces' to Spaulding's classification that do not come in contact with patients but serve as reservoir of resistant pathogens [60]. Environmental surfaces include clinical contact (medical equipment or high touch) surfaces and housekeeping surfaces. CDC defines clinical contact surfaces that can transmit infection by contaminating hands of HCWs and other patients. These surfaces includes light switches, telephones, doorknobs, beddings, X ray machines, edges of privacy curtains, walls of the toilets etc. They should be disinfected with LLDs and ILDs.

Housekeeping surfaces (wall of the patient room, floors and sinks) are rarely involved in direct spread of infection and same LLDs and ILDs can be used for decontaminating these surfaces.

For further readings of cleaning and disinfection of noncritical, semicritical and critical patient care equipments, clinical contact and housekeeping surfaces guidelines available at www.nevadaaware.com/home/GuidelinesEnvInfectControl908.pdf. may be consulted [62].

4.4.6.4. Cleaning and decontamination of specific equipment can be discussed as follows

Endoscopes : Recently, in many operative and diagnostic procedures Endoscopes are used and hence, effective decontamination is essential for patient's safety [63]. Some endoscopes are available in both flexible and rigid construction. Modern flexible fibre optic scopes (bronchoscopes, cystoscpes, gastroscopes, sigmoidoscopes etc) cannot withstand high temperatures. These are very delicate, having multiple small channels and blind ends. Hence, they are very difficult to clean and decontaminate. Endoscopes and accessories which come in contact with sterile tissue are classified as critical items and sterilization or HLD should be done ideally. Endoscopes and accessories that come in contact with mucous membrane are put into semicritical items and should be treated with HLD after use. Endoscope sterilization or HLD involve the following steps i.e. disassembling the components, cleaning and disinfection with HLD, rinsing the endoscope and its channels with sterile water to remove disinfectant, then flushing the channels with 70-90% ethyl or isopropyl alcohol and drying by forced air. Then the endoscopes are stored by hanging vertically with caps.

A logbook is to be maintained after each use and reprocessing by noting the patient's name, hospital registration number, the clinician who performed the endoscopy and HCW who did reprocessing and serial number of endoscopes etc. If any endoscope is used in a patient who has been subsequently diagnosed with CJD (Cruitzfeild Jacob disease), further follow up investigation must be done.

Ventilators : Mechanical ventilators are essentially used in Intensive Care Units (ICUs) and are common source of infection. Ventilator associated pneumonia is one of the commonest HAI after catheter associated UTI (CA-UTI). All HCWs must be trained to follow hand hygiene and use PPE while reprocessing ventilators or any other respiration devices. All disposable devices must be discarded. The ventilators should be cleaned to remove organic soil. The circuits and filters should be disposable so that it can be changed between patients.

Suction equipment : Preferably separate machine should be used for each patient. A fresh catheter must be used for every suction. After use the contents are discarded and bottle should be washed with detergent and water and then dried up. The tubing, lids, non return valve and bottles are autoclaved if required.

Dental equipments : Infection Control Practices regarding HBV and HCV are very important for dental equipments [64]. The instruments must be thoroughly cleaned before disinfection. High speed dental handpieces should be sterilized in between patients. Critical items like extraction forceps, scalpel blades, periodontal scalers etc. must be sterilised after each use. The semicritical items which come in contact with oral tissue i.e. bone amalgam condensers or syringes are sterilized and if cannot withstand heat, HLD may be done.

Ophthalmic instruments : Thorough cleaning of instruments followed by steam sterilization and if the instruments cannot withstand heat, low temperature sterilization with Ethylene oxide (EtO) can be done.

Surgical instruments : These may be cleaned manually or mechanically and sterilized [60]. Autoclaving is usually done but if the instrument is heat sensitive, low temperature sterilization with EtO can be done [60].

5. Transmission — Based additional precautions

These include airborne precautions, droplet precautions and contact precautions. These are taken when patients having or suspected of having infection with highly transmissible / epidemiologically important organism for which additional precautions are needed in addition to standard precautions [65].

Air borne pracautions : These are to be taken when patients with disease spread by droplet nuclei (<5 μm) in diameter or suspected cases are taken care of. Diseases like open/active tuberculosis, measles, chicken pox, pulmonary plague and haemorrhagic fever with pneumonia can be spread by droplet nuclei. Alongwith standard precautions the patients should be placed in a single room with negative pressure which receives ≥12 air changes per hour (≥ 12 ACH after 2001 construction). The air flow in a negative pressure room should be from outside and also should be exhausted outside but may be recirculated if the air is filtered through a High Efficiency Particulate Filter. The rooms should be closed and patients transport and movement is to be limited i.e. only when necessary. During transportation, patient must use a surgical mask to prevent dispersal of droplet nuclei. Anyone who enters the room must wear a special high filtration particulate respirator (N 95) mask.

Droplet Precautions : These are taken for large particles droplets (>5 μm diameter) and the diseases transmitted are pneumonias, pertusis, diphtheria, influenza type B, mumps and meningitis. The patient is placed in a single room or in a room with another patient infected by same agent. Surgical mask should be used by HCWs and during transportation patient should put a surgical mask.

Contact precautions : These are used to prevent transmission of antibiotic resistant bacteria, enteric infections and skin infections. HCWs must use gloves and gowns. The movement and transportation of patient should be limited.

Patient placement : Adequate spacing is required to prevent transmission of HAI. Optimum spacing between beds is 1 – 2 meters. Single room with hand washing facilities with attached toilet and bathroom is preferable to reduce transmission.

Environmental Management Practices : Safe drinking water supply, appropriate cleaning practices, housekeeping practices, laundry, pest control (mice, rodents etc) appropriate waste management facilities must be ensured to reduce HAIs. In isolation rooms, food should be served on disposable crockery and cutlery.

6. Infection control precautions in special situation

6.1. Sever Acute Respiratory Syndrome (SARS)

SARS is caused by a novel coronavirus – SARS Co – V [66] which could be found in sputum, tears, blood, urine and faeces. The virus is predominantly transmitted through droplets discharged during coughing, sneezing and talking by the patient.

Both Standard precautions and additional precautions are to be taken to prevent transmission. The patient must be placed in a single room and PPE must be used by all HCWs giving patient care, cleaning staffs, all laboratory staffs and sterilizing service workers. All waste from a SARS patient room should be treated as infectious waste. The specimens from a SARS patient should be transported in a leak proof bag (i.e. a plastic biohazard specimen bag). All infection control precautions must be followed while caring for SARS patient. A post mortem examination of SARS patient or probably having SARS is a very high risk procedure and should be avoided if possible. Staffs of the mortuary or funeral care home must be informed that the deceased had SARS. Embleming is not recommended. Even the preparation of the deceased should be discouraged.

6.2. HIV

The risk of acquiring HIV infection after needle stick or sharps injury is less than 0.5% [67]. Standard precautions using PPE and proper disposal systems for needles and sharps should be followed. The HCWs should be trained in safe sharps practices. The serological testing of patients must be done as early as possible if there is needle prick or injury by sharps. Post exposure prophylaxis should be started according to National guidelines.

6.3. HBV and HCV

For HBV and HCV same precautions and infection control practices has to be followed as HIV. All HCWs at risk of exposure to HBV must be vaccinated. No post exposure therapy to HCV is available but seroconversion of HCWs must be documented. For occupational exposure to blood borne pathogens, counselling and clinical and serological follow up must be provided.

6.4. Tuberculosis

HCWs have varying risks for exposure to tuberculosis. Multidrug resistant tuberculosis (MDR - TB) arises in countries where tuberculosis control is poor and increased incidence of HIV infection because of HIV/TB co-infection. As for infection control measure rapid detection and treatment of tuberculosis is to be done. Standard Precaution and additional airborne precaution is to be followed. During transportation, patient must wear surgical masks.

HCWs working in areas such as chest clinic, bronchoscopy unit, radiology unit, TB laboratories are at greater risk of occupational exposure to TB and MDR - TB. Hence, they have to follow Infection Control Practices.

Viral haemorrhagic fevers : Viral haemorrhagic fevers include Ebola, Marburg virus disease etc. The case fatality rate of Marburg virus disease is 25% whereas with Ebola virus 50 – 90% case fatality occur [67].

Human to human transmission occurs by direct contact with infected blood, secretions, organs, semen, even vomitus of the patient etc. Standard precautions, isolation precautions, and additional precautions are to be followed.

7. Multidrug resistant organisms and infection control practices

The multidrug resistant organisms are prevalent in Health care set up now a days because of overuse and misuse of antimicrobials. The empirical use of antimicrobials in health care set up has to be stopped and must be guided by antibiotic sensitivity test with proper dosage schedule.

In every health care set up, an antimicrobial use committee should be there, which establishes prescribing policies, audits antibiotic use etc. Antimicrobial use committee may be a subcommittee of HICC or an independent committee working hands in hands with HICC.

Transmission of MRSA, Vancomycin Resistant Enterococci (VRE) occurs through hands of HCWs, hence, transfer of staffs and patients should be reduced. Early detection of cases and placing MRSA/VRE/MDRO infected patients in a single room or in a large ward putting all MRSA infected patients (cohorting). The operating surgeons should not do surgeries until declared negative for carriage of MRSA / MDRO. Early detection of the organism and measures for managing any outbreak especially in nurseries and postoperative wards should be planned.

The same strategy has to be adopted for ESBL, AmpC β – lactamase and MBL producing Gram negative organisms.

All HCWs and patient's visitors strictly follow standard and contact precautions.

8. Biomedical waste management

Biomedical waste is defined as any waste generated during diagnosis, treatment or immunization of human beings or animals or in research activity. Hospital waste include biological or nonbiological waste, which is a reservoir of pathogenic microorganisms and require safe and reliable handling and disposal. The risk of transmitting infection is maximum with sharps contaminated with blood [68]. The steps to be followed in biomedical waste management are: generation, segregation, collection, transport, storage, treatment and final disposal.

The basic principle of Hospital waste management is to segregate hazardous and nonhazardous waste. The clinical waste (infectious) is subclassified into sharps or nonsharps. About 75 – 90% of biomedical waste is nonhazardous and 10 – 25% is hazardous. Sharps should be discarded in puncture proof containers with covers. The Govt. of India under the provision of the Environmental Act 1986, notified the Bio – Medical Waste (Management and handling) (second amendment) Rules 2000 [69]. The biomedical waste are classified into Category 1 to 10 which are segregated at source in any Health care set up. After categorization, wastes are to be put in colour coded plastic bags like yellow, red and black. The waste bags should be tied once filled to ¾ th of their capacity and should be labeled with appropriate biohazard symbol or cytotoxic waste symbol etc. On all the bags, the labels with information on the point of generation must be pasted.

Infectious nonsharp waste should be put in yellow bags which include soiled dressing, microbiology waste, cotton etc. and then incineration or deep burial is to be done. The deep burial should be 2 – 3 meters deep and atleast 1.5 meters above the ground water table.

Except anatomical waste red bags may be needed for nonsharp waste if autoclaving/microwaving/chemical treatment followed by landfill is the option (Red bags should not be incinerated as red colour contains cadmium which cause toxic emissions. Plastic disposable items e.g. gloves, catheters and i.v. sets should be put into blue/white transparent bags for shredding and disinfection before disposal by landfill. Sharps (syginges, needles, scalpel blades) should be discarded in blue/white transluscent puncture proof container). Needles should not be recapped or bent by hand. Needle should be destroyed in a needle destroying machine. Sharps are then subjected to autoclaving/microwaving/chemical treatment/shredding.

Incineration ash and solid chemical waste such as discarded medicines should be collected in black bags for disposal in secured landfill [69].

9. Surveillance of Hospital Acquired Infections(HAI)

The rates of HAI serve as indicators of quality and safety of patient care at the Health care facility. The Hospital infection Surveillance system is for early detection of outbreaks or appearance of a new organism or new MDRO or even new antimicrobial resistant organism. Surveillance should be done at hospital level and at Regional or National level.

The most commonly utilized sources of surveillance are Microbiology reports and are part of 'alert organism surveillance'. The methods are mainly daily analysis of Microbiology reports, laboratory records and clinical assessment, infection prevalence, HAI incidence study, targeted surveillance etc [70].

9.1. Calculation of rate of infection

This can be estimated by Prevalence rate, Incidence rate, Attack rate (cumulative incidence rate), Antimicrobial resistance rate (no. of MRSA/100 admissions) and incidence rate (MRSA/1000 patient days). Prompt feedback to clinicians and HCWs is most essential part to reduce the incidence of HAI and to identify the areas for improvement in quality patient care. Even molecular methods can be adopted for typing and early detection like Restriction fragment length polymorphism (RFLP), Multilocus sequence typing (MLST) etc.

In case of outbreak, the immediate control measures should be undertaken to break the chain of transmission. The control measures including, isolation or cohorting of infected case, strict hand washing and aseptic practices should be immediately implemented. Follow up of patients both clinically and Microbilogically should be done, in any outbreak.

Time to time uptodate information must be given to hospital administration, public health authorities, district, state and National Health bodies. In the final report, the cause of outbreak whether facilities available for detection of causative organisms in health care set up, measures taken to control out break and contribution of each member in Infection Control Team should be mentioned in detail.

Major outbreak generally occurs in Health Care set up due to Staphylococcus aureus/MRSA/Pseudomonas aeruginosa in NICU, or Salmonella sp. in any wards or MRSA/ESBL producing MDRO or MBL producing Pseudomonas aeruginosa/Carbapenem resistant Enterobacteriaceae in OTICU or Post operative ward etc. need special attention.

9.2. Surveillance of infections in HCWs

Surveillance in HCWs is specially required for blood borne pathogens e.g. HIV, HCV and tuberculosis, detection of carrier stage for Salmonella typhi in kitchen staffs or surgeons/residents/HCWs working in OT/Post operative wards/different ICUs should be screened for throat or nasal carriage of Staphylococcus aureus especially MRSA.

9.3. Antibiotic policy

Every health care set up must have its own antibiotic policy and a system for monitoring of antibiotic prescription

10. Routine monitoring of health care set up

Though for developed countries it is said that routine monitoring of Hospital Environment e.g. bacteriological sampling of air, floor or surfaces is not required unless and until there is

http://dx.doi.org/10.5772/55029

an outbreak. But we have experienced that routine monitoring of OT specially for Clostridium perfringens and Clostridium tetani has reduced tetanus and gas gangrene in post operative patients to actually zero in our hospital.

We collect minimum 5 swabs for each OT from the sites like 1. OT table, 2. Overhead lamp, 3. Boyle's apparatus, 4. Instrument trolly, 5. Floor near OT table routinely on Monday morning. After fumigation on Saturdays and closing the OT for 40 - 48 hours about 80 – 100 swabs on every Monday morning are collected. With proper cleaning of wound and implementing all aseptic practices, no tetanus or gas gangrene cases have been reported in last 10 years, even from Trauma ICU and Emergency OTs where Road accident cases are handled. Moreover, our Infection Control Nurse, collect swab from different wards and ICUs from 5 minimum sites and maximum 10 sites e.g. 1. Disinfectant solution, 2. Dressing trolly, 3. IV stand, 4. Fabric, 5. Switch Board, 6. Gauge Piece, 7. O2 Cylinder, 8. Ventilator 9. Suction machine, 10. Gown.

On every Tuesday, approximately 50 – 80 swabs, moistened with Brain Heart Infusion broth are collected from those above mentioned sites and cultured on Nutrient agar and then incubated at 37^0C overnight. Colony counts and detection of organisms are done by Infection Control Technician and Microbiologists in the Infection Control Team. Disinfectant solutions where cheatle forceps are kept and gauze pieces which are used in dressings, eye drop from ophthalmology wards, pads from Labour room and Gynaecology & Obstetric wards are compulsorily taken for monitoring. If any organism is grown from disinfectant solution, gauze pieces or eye drops, immediately the clinician and ward sister is informed telephonically to discard it. Though our hospital is a tertiary care hospital but it is in a rural set up and caters patients from different nearby villages also. By observing this protocol, major outbreaks in Ophthalmology or Post operative wards could be reduced to almost nil in last 10 years.

10.1. Hospital infection report form

Every Health care set up must have their own Hospital infection Report form The Hospital infection report form must include name of the patient, age & sex, registration number, laboratory number, date of admission, bed number, ward, name of the clinician, clinical diagnosis, history of any major invasive procedure or operation (date/OT used/duration of ICU stay), nature of infection, antibiotics received etc. The form should be filled up by clinician, sent to Microbiology laboratory and informed to Infection Control Team.

11. Educational programmes for hospital staffs

We also take different educational programmes like CMEs and Workshops for HCWs, technitians and doctors from time to time about infection control practices e.g. hand hygiene, antimicrobial resistance, sterilization of OT etc.

The only silver lining to the serious problem of HAI is 36% of all HAIs are preventable if Infection Control Practices are followed by HCWs. Hand hygiene is the simplest and most effective measure before and after each patient contact to reduce the risk of HAI.

12. Team work

Infact, Infection control in any Health care set up is a team work. Each and every staff involved in patient care should take part in Infection Control Programme, then only Infection Control Programme can run successfully.

Author details

Silpi Basak, Monali N. Rajurkar, Sanjay K. Mallick and Ruchita O. Attal

Department of Microbiology J.N. Medical College Wardha (M.S.), India

References

[1] Selwy, S. Hospital infection: The first 2500 years J.Hosp Infect (1991). Suppl.A):, 5-64.

[2] In Hospital- acquired infections: guidelines for controlGovt of India (Deptt. Of Health), Nirmal Bhavan, New Delhi- 110011, (1992).

[3] Emori, T. G, Culver, D. H, Horan, T. C, et al. National nosocomial infections surveillance system (NNIS) : description of surveillance methods. Am. J. Infect. Control (1991)., 19, 19-35.

[4] Brachman, P. S. Epidemiology of Nosocomial infections. In: Bennet JV, Brachman PS, eds Hospital infections. Philadelphia : Lippincott. Raven, (1998)., 1998, 3-16.

[5] Centers for Disease Control; health care associated infectionshttp://www.cdc.gov/ncidod/dhqp/healthDis.html(2006).

[6] Ostrowsky, B. Epidemiology of Healthcare- Associated Infections In: Bennet and Brachman's Hospital infections. Jewris WR ed. Philadelphia: Lippincott Williams & Wlkin;(2007)., 2007, 3-24.

[7] WHO: Guidelines on Prevention and Control of Hospital Associated InfectionsWorld Health Organization. South East Asian Region. Geneva : WHO;(2002).

[8] Kim, J. M, Park, E. S, Jeong, J. S, et al. Multicenter Surveillance study for nosocomial infections in major hospitalsin Korea. Nosocomial Infection Surveillance Committee of the Korean Society for Nosocomial infection Control Am J. Infect Control.(2000)., 28, 454-458.

[9] Klevens, M. R, Edwards, J. R, Richards, J. C. L, Horan, T. C, Gaynes, R. P, Pollock, D. A, & Cardo, D. M. (2007). Estimating health care-associated infections and deaths in U.S. hospitals, 2002. Public Health Rep, , 122, 160-166.

[10] World Health Organization ((2011). Report on the burden of endemic health care- associated infections worldwide. WHO Document Production Services, 978-9-24150-150-7Geneva.

[11] Mukharjee, V. Nosocomial infections in India: Assuming dangerous proportions, internet Google search.

[12] Childs, D. Hospital Infections Kill More than Cors. AIDS and Breast Cancer. Available at: http://www.rense.general741hosp.htm.

[13] Vincent, J. L. Nosocomial infections in adult intensive care units Lancet (2003). , 361, 2068-2077.

[14] Washington CW JrStephen DA, Williams MJ, Elmer WK, Gary WP, Paul CS, Gail LW. Introduction to Microbiology Chapter 1 In: Koneman;s Colour Atlas and Textbook of Diagnostic Microbiology, 6th ed, Lippincott Williams & Wilkins, Philadelphia PA, USA, (2006). , 1-66.

[15] Siegel, J. D, Rhinehart, E, Jackson, M, & Chiarell, O. L. The Healthcare Infection Control Practices Advisory Committee Guideline for Isolation Precautions: Preventing Transmission of Infectious Agents in Healthcare settings. Atlanta GA: Centers for Disease Control and Prevention, (2007). Available at: http://www.cdc.gov/ncidod/dhqp/pdf/isolationn2007.pdf.

[16] Garner, J. S. Guideline for isolation precautions in hospitals. The Hospital Infection Control Practices Advisory committee. Infect Control Hosp Epidemiol (1996). , 17, 53-80.

[17] Lockhart, S. R, Abramson, M. A, & Beekmann, S. E. Antimicrobial resistance among Gram negative bacilli causing infections in intensive care unit patients in the United States between 1993 and 2004. J.Clin.Microbiol. (2007). , 45(10), 3352-3359.

[18] Falagas, M. E, & Karageorgopoulos, D. E. Pandrug resistance (PDR), Extensive drug resistance (XDR) and Multidrug resistance (MDR) among Gram Negative Bacilli : Need for international Harmonization in Terminology. Clin.Inf.Diseases. (2008). , 48, 1121-22.

[19] Peterson, L. R. Bad bugs, no drugs, no ESCAPE revisited Clin.Infect.Dis. (2009). , 49(6), 992-993.

[20] Gupta, E, Mohanty, S, Sood, S, Dhawan, B, Das, B. K, & Kapil, A. Emerging resistance to carbapenems in a tertiary care hospital in north India. Indian J Med Res July (2006). , 124, 95-8.

[21] Basak, S, Khodke, M, Bose, S, & Mallick, S. K. Inducible AmpC Beta-Lactamase Producing Pseudomonas Aeruginosa Isolated In a rural Hospital of Central India. Journal of Clinical and Diagnostic Research. (2009).

[22] Attal, R. O, Basak, S, Mallick, S. K, & Bose, S. Metallobetalactamase Producing Pseudomonas aeruginosa: An emerging Threat To Clinicians Journal of Clinical and Diagnostic Research. (2010).

[23] Gould, C. V, Umscheid, C. A, Agrawal, R. K, et al. HI.AAC/CDC Guideline for Prevention of Catheter. Associated Urinary Tract Infection. HICPAC, (2009). Available at: http://www.cdc.gov.nhsn/pdfs/pscManual/tpscCAUTIcurrent.pdf.

[24] Richards, M, Edwards, J, Culver, D, & Gaynes, R. Nosocomial infections in medical intensive care units in the United States. National Nosocomial Infections Surveillance System. Crit Care Med. (1999)., 27, 887-892.

[25] Warren, J. W. Nosocomial urinary tract infections. In Mandell GL, Bennett JE, Dolin R (eds), Principles and Practice of Infectious Diseases. 6th ed. Philadelphia, PA: Elsevier Churchill Livingstone, (2005).

[26] Tablan, O. C, Anderson, L. J, Besser, R, et al. Guidelines for preventing health care associated pneumonia: Recommendations of CDC and the Healthcare Infection control Practices Advisory Committee 2003. Morb Mort Weekly Rep. (2004). RR-3):1-36.

[27] Fiel, S. Guidelines and Critical pathways for severe hospital- acquired pneumonia. Chest, (2001)., 119, 412-418.

[28] ATS Board of Directors and IDSA Guideline CommitteeGuidelines for the management of adults with hospital- acquired ventilator associated and health care- associated pneumonia. Am. J. Respir. Crit Care med (2005).

[29] Mangram, A. J, et al. Guideline for prevention of surgical site infection, 1999. Hospital infection Control Practices Advisory Committee. Infection Control and Hospital Epidemiology. (1999)., 20(4), 250-278.

[30] Harrop, J. S, Styliaras, J. C, Ooi, Y. C, et al. Contributing factors to Surgical site infections. J.A.Acad. Orthop.Surg. February (2012).

[31] Horan, T. C, et al. CDC definitions of nosocomial surgical site infections 1992: a modification of CDC definitions of surgical wound infections. American Journal of Infection Control. (1992)., 20(5), 271-274.

[32] Kirkland, K, Briggs, J, Trivette, S, et al. The impact of surgical site infections in the 1990s: attributable mortality, excess length of hospitalization and extra costs. Infect Control Hosp Epidemiol. (1999)., 20, 725-730.

[33] Rosenthal, V. D, Maki, D. G, Salomao, R, et al. Device- associated nosocomial infections in 55 intensive care units of 8 developing countries. Ann. Intern med. (2006)., 145, 582-591.

[34] Siegle, J. D. The newborn nursery and the neonatal intensive care unit. Ch. 25 In Bennet and Brachmans Hospital infections Jewris WR ed. Philadelphia: Lippincott Williams & Wlkin;(2007)., 2007, 417-445.

[35] Mallick, S, Basak, S, & Bose, S. Inducible Clindamycin resistance in Staphylococcus aureus A therapeutic challenge Journal of Clinical & diagnostic Research June (2009).

[36] Mallick, S, & Basak, S. MRSA- too many hurdles to overcome : a study from Central India, Tropical Doctor, (2010). , 40(2), 108-110.

[37] Clinical and Laboratory Standards Institute(2006). Performance standards for antimicrobial disk tests; Approved Standards, 9th ed. CLSI Document M2- M9, Wayne PA., 26(1)

[38] Mallick, S, & Basak, S. Accurate detection of methicillin- resistant Staphylococcus aureus in day to day practice : a great help to clinicians, J. Indian Med. Assoc. (2011). , 109, 892-5.

[39] Basak, S, & Deshpande, M. M. A study of Methicillin Resistant Staphylococcus aureus (MRSA) isolated in a rural Medical College, Indian Medical Gazette (1997). CXXXI;, 304-6.

[40] Basak, S, Attal, R. O, & Rajurkar, M. N. Pseudomonas Aeruginosa And Newer β-Lactamases:An Emerging Resistance Threat. In: Infection Control- Update, edited by Christopher Sudhakar, Intech publication, February (2012). Online open access book)http://www.intechopen.com/articles/show/title/pseudomonas-aeruginosa-and-newer-lactamases-an-emerging-resistance-threat, 2012, 181-198.

[41] Carter, M. W, Oakton, K. J, Warner, M, & Livermore, D. M. (2000). Detection of extended spectrum beta lactamases in Klebsiellae with the Oxoid combination disk method. J Clin Microbiol. , 38, 4228-4232.

[42] Washington CW JrStephen DA., Williams MJ., Elmer WK., Gary WP., Paul CS., Gail LW. ((2006). Antimicrobial Susceptibility Testing chapter 17 In Koneman's Colour Atlas and Textbook of Diagnostic Microbiology, 6th ed, Lippincott Williams & Wilkins, 100781730147PA, USA., 945-1021.

[43] Yagi, T, Wachino, J, Kurokawa, H, Suzuki, S, et al. (2005). Practical methods using boronic acid compounds for identification of class C β-lactamase producing Klebsiella pneumoniae and Escherichia coli. J of Clin Microbiol. , 43(6), 2551-2558.

[44] Lee, K, Chong, Y, Shin, H B, Kim, Y A, Yong, D, & Yum, J H. (2001). Modified Hodge and EDTA disk synergy test to screen metallobetalactamases producing strains of Pseudomonas spp and Acinetobacter spp. Clin Microbiol Infect. , 7, 88-91.

[45] Yong, D, Lee, K, Yum, J H, & Shin, H B. Rossolinism, Chong Y. ((2002). Imipenem-EDTA disk method for differentiation of metallobetalactamases producing clinical isolates of Pseudomonas spp and Acinetobacter spp. J Clin Microbiol. , 40, 3798-3801.

[46] Walsh, T. R, Bolmstrom, A, Qwarnstrom, A, & Gales, . . (2002). Evaluation of a new Etest for detecting metall-lactamases in routine clinical testing. J. Clin. Microbiol. Vol 40 pp. (2755-2759).

[47] Basak, S, Rajurkar, M. N, Attal, R. O, & Mallick, S. K. Intensive Care Unit : A breeding ground for antibiotic resistant bacteria, International Journal of Clinical Research and Review (2012).

[48] Practical Guidelines for Infection Control in Health Care Facilities SEARO regional publication number 41 WPRO regional publicationWorld Health Organization, (2004).

[49] Labarraque, A. G. In: Porter J (ed.) Instructions and Observations Regarding the Use of the chlorides of soda and lime. New Haven, CT: Baldwin and Treaddway, (1829). French).

[50] Semmelweis, I. Etiology and Concept Prophylaxis of Childbed Fever (trans. Carter KC), 1st ed. Medison WI: The University of Wisconsin Press, (1983).

[51] Magiorakos, A. P, Suetens, C, Boyd, L, et al. National hand hygiene campaigns in Europe, Euro Survell, (2009). Available at: http://www.eurosurveillance.org/images/dynamics/EE/VV14N17/art19190.pdf., 2000-2009.

[52] World Health OrganizationGuide to Implementation of the WHO Multi model Hand Hygiene Improvement Strategy. Available at: http://www.who.int/patientsafety/en/.

[53] Kilpatrick, C, Allegranzi, B, & Pittet, D. The global impact of hand hygiene campaigning. Euro Survell, (2009). Available at: http://www.eurosurveillance.org/images/dynamic/EE/art1919.pdf.

[54] Trampuz, A, & Widmer, A. F. Hand Hygiene: A frequently missed lifesaving opportunity during patient care. Mayo Clin Proc. (2004)., 79, 109-116.

[55] Pittet, D, Mourouga, P, & Perneger, T. V. Compliance with hand washing in a teaching hospital: Infection control program. Ann Intern med, (1999)., 130, 126-130.

[56] Kampf, G, & Kramer, A. Epidemiologic background of hand hygiene and evaluation of the most important agents for scrubs and rubs. Clin Microbiol Rev. (2004)., 17(4), 863-893.

[57] World Heal OrganizationWHO Guidelines on Hand Hygiene in Health Care. First Global Patient Safety Challenge. Clean Care is Safer Care. Available at: http://www.who.int/patientsafety/en/.

[58] Widemer, A. F, & Frei, R. Decontamination, disinfection and sterilization. In: Murray TR, Baron EJ, Jorgensen JH, Plater MA, Yolkan RH (eds) Manual of Clinical Microbiology, 8th ed. Washington DC:ASM Press, (2003).

[59] Siegel, J. D, Rhinehart, E, Jackson, M, & Chiarello, L. The Healthcare Infection Control Practices Advisory Committee Guideline for isolation Precautions: Preventing Transmission of infectious AAgents in Healthcare Settings 2007. Atlanta GA: Centers for Disease Control and Prevention, (2007). Available at: http://www.cdc.gov/ncidod/dhqp/pdf/isolation2007.pdf.

[60] Rutala, W. A, & Weber, D. J. The Healthcare Infection Control practices Advisory Committee (HICPAC). Guideline for Disinfection and Sterilization Healthcare Facilities. Atlanta GA:CDC;(2008).

[61] Spaulding, E. H. Chemical disinfection of medical and surgical materials. In: Lawrence C, Block SS (eds.) Disinfection, Sterilization and Presevation. Philadelphia, PA:Lea & Febiger, (1968)., 1968, 517-531.

[62] GuidelinesAvailable at: www.nevadaaware.com/home/GuidelinesEnvInfectControl908.pdf.

[63] Nelson, D. B, Jarvis, W. R, Rutala, W. A, et al. Multi society guideline for reprocessing flexible endoscopes. Society for Healthcare Epidemiology of America. Infect Control Hosp Epidemiol. (2003)., 24(7), 532-537.

[64] Gurevich, I, Dubin, R, & Cunha, B. A. Dental instrument and device sterilization and disinfection practices. J. Hosp. Infect.(1996)., 32(4), 295-304.

[65] World Health OrganizationGuidelines on Prevention and Control Hospital Associated Infections. World Health Organization. South East Asian Region. Geneva, Switzerland: World Health Organization, (2002).

[66] Wenzel, R. P, & Edmond, M. B. Listening to SARS: Lessons for infection control. Annals of Internal Medicine. (2003). Oct.7;, 139(7), 592-3.

[67] Chin, J. editor. Control of communicable diseases manual. 17th ed. Washington DC, American Public Health Association, (2000).

[68] World Health OrganizationPrevention of hospital acquired infections- A practical guide. 2nd ed. Geneva: WHO,(2002). Document no. WHO/CDS/EPH/2002.12. Electronic access: http://whqlibdoc.who.int/hq/2002/WHO_CDS_CSR_EPH_2002.12.pdf.

[69] Biomedical Waste (Management and Handling)(Second amendment) Rules (2000). Ministry of Environmental and Forest Notification, New Delhi, the 2nd June 2000.

[70] Ducel, G, & Fabry, J. Nicolle L (eds). Prevention of Hospital Acquired Infections. A Practical Guide, 2nd ed. Geneva: World Health Organization, (2002).

Section 2

Emerging Trends of HAI

Chapter 2

Pseudomonas aeruginosa: Multi-Drug-Resistance Development and Treatment Options

Georgios Meletis and Maria Bagkeri

Additional information is available at the end of the chapter

http://dx.doi.org/10.5772/55616

1. Introduction

Antibiotic resistance is a worldwide problem of major importance. Isolations in some countries of multi-drug-resistant (resistant to three or more classes of antimicrobials), extensively-drug-resistant (resistant to all but one or two classes) or even pan-drug-resistant (resistant to all available classes) Gram-negative pathogens are causing therapeutic problems and- in the same time- are posing infection control issues in many hospitals. In fact, numerous studies highlight the link between multi-drug-resistance and increased morbidity and mortality, increased length of hospital stay and higher hospital costs [1-4].

Pseudomonas aeruginosa is a Gram-negative opportunistic nosocomial pathogen responsible for a wide range of infections that may present high rates of antimicrobial resistance. The genome of this microorganism is among the largest in the bacterial world allowing for great genetic capacity and high adaptability to environmental changes. In fact, *P. aeruginosa* has 5567 genes encoded in 6.26 Mbp of DNA while *Escherichia coli* K12 for example has 4279 genes encoded in 4.46 Mbp and *Haemophilus influenzae* Rd has 1.83 Mbp encoding 1714 genes [5]. This large genetic armamentarium- that can be further enriched with the addition of genes acquired by transferable genetic elements via horizontal gene transfer- is a major contributing factor to its formidable ability to develop resistance against all known antibiotics.

Generally, antibiotic resistance mechanisms of *P. aeruginosa* can be divided in intrinsic and acquired. Intrinsic refers to resistance that is a consequence of a large selection of genetically-encoded mechanisms and acquired refers to resistance that is achieved via the acquisition of additional mechanisms or is a consequence of mutational events under selective pressure.

2. Intrinsic resistance of *Pseudomonas aeruginosa*

P. aeruginosa shows inherent resistance to antimicrobial agents through a variety of mechanisms: (1) decreased permeability of the outer membrane, (2) efflux systems which actively pump antibiotics out of the cell, and (3) production of antibiotic-inactivating enzymes [6].

2.1. Outer membrane permeability

The outer membrane of Gram-negative bacteria is a barrier which prevents large hydrophilic molecules to pass through it. Aminoglycosides and colistin interact with lipopolysaccharides changing the permeability of the membrane in order to pass whereas beta-lactams and quinolones need to diffuse through certain porin channels.

Bacteria produce two major classes of porins: general; which allow almost any hydrophilic molecule to pass [7] and specific; which have binding sites for certain molecules, allowing them to be oriented and pass in the most energy-efficient way [8].

Most bacteria posses lots of general porins and relatively few specific ones. However, the exact opposite occurs for *P. aeruginosa* that expresses mainly specific porins [7].

2.2. Efflux systems

P. aeruginosa expresses several efflux pumps that expel drugs together with other substances out of the bacterial cell. These pumps consist of three proteins: (1) a protein transporter of the cytoplasmatic membrane that uses energy in the form of proton motive force, (2) a periplasmic connective protein, and (3) an outer membrane porin [5].

Most antibiotics- except polymyxins- are pumped out [9,10] by these efflux systems (Table 1) therefore their first two components are named multidrug efflux (Mex) along with a letter (e.g. MexA and MexB). The outer membrane porin is called Opr along with a letter (e.g. OprM) [11].

2.3. Antibiotic-inactivating enzymes

P. aeruginosa belongs to the SPICE group of bacteria (*Serratia* spp., *P. aeruginosa,* Indole positive *Proteus, Citrobacter* spp., *Enterobacter* spp.). These microorganisms share a common characteristic: the ability to produce chromosomal-encoded and inducible AmpC beta-lactamases. These are cephalosporinases that hydrolyze most beta-lactams and are not inhibited by the beta lactamase inhibitors.

Another endogenous beta-lactamase produced by *P. aeruginosa* is the class D oxacillinase PoxB [12,13]. This enzyme however has only been found in laboratory mutants and is not clinically significant.

http://dx.doi.org/10.5772/55616

Efflux system	Efflux pump family	Substrates	References
MexAB-OprM	Resistance Nodulation Division (RND)	Fluoroquinolones Aminoglycosides β-Lactams (preferably Meropenem, Ticarcillin) Tetracycline Tigecycline Chloramphenicol	[17]
MexCD-OprJ	Resistance Nodulation Division (RND)	Fluoroquinolones β-Lactams (preferably Meropenem, Ticarcillin) Tetracycline Tigecycline Chloramphenicol Erythromycin Roxythromycin	[17]
MexEF-OprN	Resistance Nodulation Division (RND)	Fluoroquinolones β-Lactams (preferably Meropenem, Ticarcillin) Tetracycline Tigecycline Chloramphenicol	[17] [18]
MexXY-OprM	Resistance Nodulation Division (RND)	Fluoroquinolones Aminoglycosides β-Lactams (preferably Meropenem, Ticarcillin, Cefepime) Tetracycline Tigecycline Chloramphenicol	[17]
AmrAB-OprA	Resistance Nodulation Division (RND)	Aminoglycosides	[19]
PmpM	Multidrug And Toxic compound Extrusion (MATE)	Fluoroquinolones	[17]
Mef(A)	Major Facilitator Superfamily (MFS)	Macrolides	[20]
$ErmE_{PAF}$	Small Multidrug Resistance (SMR)	Aminoglycosides	[21]

Table 1. Efflux systems of *P. aeruginosa*.

3. Antipseudomonal treatment

Despite the intrinsic resistance of *P. aeruginosa* to many antimicrobials, some antibiotics are active against this microorganism [14]. Those used more frequently belong to three antibiotic classes: (1) Beta-lactams, (2) Quinolones and (3) Aminoglycosides (Table 2).

3.1. Beta-lactams

Beta-lactams bind to and inactivate penicillin-binding proteins (PBPs) that are transpeptidases involved in bacterial cell wall synthesis [15]. The group of beta-lactam antibiotics includes penicillins, cepholosporins, monobactams and carbapenems. The beta-lactams that are most active against *P. aeruginosa* are: Piperacillin and ticarcillin (penicillins), ceftazidime (3rd generation cephalosporin), cefepime (4th generation cephalosporin), aztreonam (monobactam), imipenem, meropenem and doripenem (carbapenems).

3.2. Quinolones

Quinolones are synthetic antimicrobials that block DNA replication by inhibiting the activity of DNA gyrase and topoisomerase IV [16]. The fluorquinolones with anti-pseudomonal activity are ciprofloxacin, levofloxacin and ofloxacin.

Antibiotic Class	Mechanism of action	Drug
Penicillins	Bacterial cell wall synthesis inhibition	Ticarcillin
Penicillin / Beta-lactamase inhibitor	Bacterial cell wall synthesis inhibition	Ticarcillin/Clavulanic acid
		Piperacillin/Tazobactam
Cefalosporins	Bacterial cell wall synthesis inhibition	Ceftazidime
		Cefepime
Monobactams	Bacterial cell wall synthesis inhibition	Aztreonam
Carbapenems	Bacterial cell wall synthesis inhibition	Imipenem
		Meropenem
		Doripenem
Fluoroquinolones	Block of DNA synthesis	Ciprofloxacin
		Levofloxacin
		Ofloxacin
Aminoglycosides	Protein synthesis inhibition	Gentamycin
		Tobramycin
		Amikacin

Table 2. Commonly used anti-pseudomonal drugs.

http://dx.doi.org/10.5772/55616

3.3. Aminoglycosides

Aminoglycosides inhibit protein synthesis by binding to the 30S or 50S ribosomal subunit [22]. Drugs of this antibiotic class that can be used against *P. aeruginosa* are tobramycin, amikacin and gentamicin. Aminoglycosides are associated with ototoxicity and nefrotoxicity [23]. Because of these adverse effects and because of their narrow therapeutic range, aminoglycosides are used in combination with agents belonging to other antibiotic classes. The only treatment in which aminoglycosides are recommended as monotherapy is that of urinary tract infections due to *P. aeruginosa* [14].

4. Acquired resistance of *Pseudomonas aeruginosa*

Apart from being resistant to a variety of antimicrobial agents, *P. aeruginosa* develops resistance to anti-pseudomonal drugs as well. This acquired resistance is a consequence of mutational changes or the acquisition of resistance mechanisms via horizontal gene transfer and can occur during chemotherapy [24]. Mutational events may lead to over-expression of endogenous beta-lactamases or efflux pumps, diminished expression of specific porins and target site modifications while acquisition of resistance genes mainly refers to transferable beta-lactamases and aminoglycoside-modifying enzymes (Table 3).

Resistance to	Resistance mechanism
Beta-lactams	Endogenous beta-lactamases
	Acquired beta-lactamases
	Efflux
	Diminished permeability
Fluoroquinolones	Target site mutations
	Efflux
Aminoglycosides	Aminoglycoside-modifying enzymes
	Efflux
	16S rRNA methylases
Polymyxins	LPS modification

Table 3. Resistance mechanisms of *P. aeruginosa* to anti-pseudomonal drugs.

4.1. Resistance to beta-lactams

Resistance to beta-lactam antibiotics is multi-factorial but is mediated mainly by inactivating enzymes called beta-lactamases. These enzymes cleave the amide bond of the beta-lactam ring causing antibiotic inactivation and are classified according to a structural [25] and a functional [26] classification.

Among the beta-lactams, carbapenems are the most efficient against *P. aeruginosa*. These agents are stable to the hydrolytic effect of the majority of the beta-lactamases including the Extended Spectrum Beta-Lactamases (ESBLs) [27]. For this reason, the enzymes that possess carbapenemase activity, namely the carbapenemases [28], will be discussed separately in this section.

4.1.1. Expression of endogenous beta-lactamases

Resistance to beta-lactams in clinical isolates is commonly due to the presence of AmpC beta-lactamases [29-36]. Furthermore, the production of AmpC beta-lactamases in *P. aeruginosa* can be induced by a number of beta-lactam antibiotics such as benzyl penicillines, narrow spectrum cephalosporins and imipenem [37]. In fact, this mutational derepression is one of the most common mechanisms of resistance to beta-lactams in *P. aeruginosa* [29,32,33,36].

AmpC enzymes are not carbapenemases, they posses however a low potential of carbapenem hydrolysis and their overproduction combined with efflux pumps over-expression and/or diminished outer membrane permeability has been proven to lead also to carbapenem resistance in *P. aeruginosa* [38].

4.1.2. Acquired beta-lactamases

Acquired beta-lactamases are typically encoded by genes which are located in transferable genetic elements such as plasmids or transposons [39] often on integrons [40-49]. Integrons are genetic elements that capture and mobilize genes [50]. Other genetic elements associated with transferable resistance in *P. aeruginosa* are the mobile insertion sequences called ISCR elements [49,51-53].

Different types of transferable beta-lactamases have been found in clinical *P. aeruginosa* isolates around the world (Table 4).

Among them, carbapenemases are of major clinical importance because they inactivate carbapenems together with other beta-lactams. Ambler class A ESBLs hydrolyze penicillins, narrow- and broad-spectrum cephalosporins and aztreonam [54]. Some TEM and SHV enzymes do not possess broad-spectrum cephalosporinase activity and are called restricted-spectrum beta-lactamases. Class D OXA beta-lactamases are a heterogenous group of enzymes and not all share the same properties. Generally, most of them show a preference for cloxacillin over benzylpenicillin. They confer resistance to amino- and carboxypenicillins and narrow – spectrum cephalosporins even though some of them are ESBLs and a few members of the class present carbapenemase activity [24].

4.1.3. Carbapenemases

P. aeruginosa is the species in which all types of transferable carbapenemases, except SIM-1 [55], have been detected. The class B carbapenemases that bear Zn^{2+} in their active center [56] are the most frequent around the world in *P. aeruginosa* isolates and are called metallo-beta-lactamases (MBLs). They hydrolyse *in vitro* all beta-lactams except aztreonam and are the major cause of high-level carbapenem resistance. Genes that encode MBLs are commonly found as

http://dx.doi.org/10.5772/55616

Ambler molecular class	Bush-Jacoby-Madeiros group	Enzymes	References
A	2b	TEM-1, -2, -90, -110, SHV-1	[57,58]
	2be	PER-1, -2 VEB-1, -2, -3 TEM-4, -21, -24, -42, -116 SHV-2a, -5, -12 GES/IBC-1, -2, -5, -8, -9 BEL LBT 802 CTX-M-1, -2, -43	[10] [53] [59-62]
	2c	PSE-1 (CARB-2), PSE-4 (CARB-1), CARB-3, CARB-4, CARB-like, AER-1	[10] [63]
	2f	KPC-2, -5	[64,65]
B	3	IMP-1, -4, -6, -7, -9, -10, -12, -13, -15, -16, -18, -22 VIM-1, -2, -3, -4, -5, -7, -8, -11, -13, -15, -16,-17, -18 SPM-1 GIM-1 AIM-1 NDM-1	[10] [47] [66-76]
C	1	AmpC	[77]
D	2d	OXA LCR-1 NPS-1	[10] [12] [54] [57] [78-80]

Table 4. Beta-lactamases found in *P. aeruginosa* isolates.

gene cassettes in integrons and are transferable [42]. Interestingly, more resistance genes for other antibiotic classes can be present in the same integrons contributing thus in the development of a multi-drug resistant phenotype.

IMP and VIM type MBLs were first identified in Japan [81] and Italy [82] respectively and have spread though all continents since then. Other metallo-enzymes are more geographically restricted. SPM-1, after causing outbreaks in Brazil [28], has been found in Basel [83] in a single isolate recovered from a patient previously hospitalized in Brazil. GIM-1 and AIM-1 were reported from Germany [41] and Australia [84] and did not spread elsewhere. Finally, the only report for NDM-1 in *P. aeruginosa* was made from Serbia [76].

Ambler class A carbapenemase KPC was first reported in *P. aeruginosa* isolates in Colombia [64] but KPC-producing *P. aeruginosa* isolates have not been reported from other continents except Latin America. KPCs present high rates of carbapenem hydrolysis and inactivate all other beta-lactams including aztreonam.

Enzymes GES/IBC belong to the same enzymatic class but their carbapenemase activity is not as high as that of the KPCs. It may become important however if combined with diminished outer membrane permeability or efflux over-expression. For *P. aeruginosa,* GES-2 has been reported in South Africa [85] and IBC-2 in Greece [86].

Class D carbapenemases like OXA-198 have been found in *P. aeruinosa* isolates although such findings are rather rare for this species [87]. The most clinically important carbapenemases are summarized in Table 5.

Ambler molecular class	Bush-Jacoby-Madeiros group	Carbapenemases
A	2f	KPC
B	3	IMP enzymes
		VIM enzymes
		SPM-1
		GIM-1
		AIM-1
		NDM-1

Table 5. Clinically important carbapenemases found in *P. aeruginosa* isolates.

4.1.4. Efflux systems over-expression

Among the various efflux systems of *P. aeruginosa,* MexAB-OprM, MexXY-OprM and MexCD-OprJ play an important role in developing beta-lactam resistance [88]. Between these three, MexAB-OprM accommodates the broadest range of beta-lactams [24], is by far the better exporter of meropenem [24] and is most frequently related to beta-lactam resistance in clinical *P. aeruginosa* isolates [33,89]. The efflux pumps may be over-expressed in some isolates [90] contributing thus, together with other mechanisms in the development of multi-drug resistance [24].

4.1.5. Diminished permeability

OprD is a specific porin of the outer membrane of *P. aeruginosa* through which carbapenems (mainly imipenem) enter into the periplasmic space [91]. Diminished expression [92] or mutational loss [93] of this porin is the most common mechanism of resistance to carbapenems [24,94] and is frequently associated with efflux pumps and/or AmpC over-expression [36,38].

Diminished expression or loss of the OprD porin is a frequent phenomenon during imipenem treatment [95].

4.2. Resistance to fluoroquinolones

High-level resistance to fluoroquinolones is mediated by target site modifications. Efflux plays a contributing role as well [96,97] and the two mechanisms often coexist [32,98-100].

4.2.1. DNA gyrase and topoisomerase IV mutations

Gyrase and topoisomerase are comprised by two subunits each. DNA gyrase (GyrA and GyrB) is the main target of fluoroquinolones in *P. aeruginosa*. Consequently, mutations are most common for this enzyme rather than for topoisomerase IV (ParC and ParE) [98-102]. Highly resistant isolates have multiple mutations in *gyrA* and/or *parC* [98,101-103] while mutations regarding the other subunits are less frequently encountered [100-102,104].

4.2.2. Efflux pumps contribution

Four efflux pumps contribute to fluoroquinolone resistance: MexAB-OprM, MexCD-OprJ, MexEF-OprN and MexXY-OprM [105] as a consequence of mutational events in their repressor genes [24]. Among these, MexAB-OprM, MexCD-OprJ, and MexEF-OprN have been associated to fluoroquinolone resistance in clinical isolates [31,105-107] whereas MexXY-OprM has only been linked rarely to such type of resistance [106].

4.3. Resistance to aminoglycosides

Acquired resistance to aminoglycosides is mediated by transferable aminoglycoside-modifying enzymes (AMEs), rRNA methylases and derepression of endogenous efflux systems [24,108,109].

4.3.1. Aminoglycoside-modifying enzymes

Modification and subsequent inactivation of aminoglycosides is achieved by three deferent mechanisms: (1) acetylation, by aminoglycoside acetyltransferases (AACs), (2) adenylation, by aminoglycoside nucleotidyltransferases (ANTs), and (3) phosphorylation, by aminoglycoside posphoryltransferases (APHs) [108].

Genes encoding AMEs are typically found on integrons together with other genes responsible for transferable resistance for other antibiotic classes. This way AMEs become important determinants for the development of multi-drug resistance in *P. aeruginosa* and other species [24,108,109].

Enzymatic families that acetylate the 3 and 6′ position of the antibiotic are the most common. Five subfamilies of AAC(3) and two of AAC(6′) have been described for *P. aeruginosa,* each one presenting different preferences for aminoglycoside substrates (Table 6).

Among the nucleotidyltransferases, ANT(2')-I is the most frequently encountered in *P. aerugiosa.* This enzyme is present in isolates showing resistance to gentamicin and tobramycin but not to amikacin [109].

Almost all phosphoryltransferases of *P. aeruginosa* act in the 3' position of the aminoglycoside molecule [24]. However, they have less clinical importance because of the fact that they inactivate aminoglycosides that are not routinely used for the treatment of *P. aeruginosa* infections such as kanamycin and neomycin [109]. The enzymes of this family that inactivate anti-pseudomonal aminoglycosides are APH(3')-VI [110-112], APH(3')-IIb-like [113] and APH(2'') [110]. Despite being reported in some cases, these enzymes remain rare for clinical *P. aeruginosa* isolates [24].

4.3.2. Efflux systems

Resistance to aminoglycosides in *P. aeruginosa* can occur independently of aminoglycoside-modifying enzymes in cystic fibrosis patients. This type of resistance has been reported in several studies [99,118-120] and is attributable to over-expression of the MexXY-OprM efflux pump.

4.3.3. 16S rRNA methylases

Methylation of the 16S rRNA of the A site of the 30S ribosomal subunit interferes with aminoglycoside binding and consequently promotes high-level resistance to all aminoglycosides [24]. Different 16S rRNA methylases have been described for *P. aeruginosa*: RmtA [112,121], RmtB [122], ArmA [122,123] and RmtD which is commonly found together with the MBL SPM-1 in Brazil [124,125].

5. Treatment options for MDR *Pseudomonas aeruginosa*

Different combinations of the aforementioned mechanisms may be present in a single *P. aeruginosa* isolate leading to simultaneous resistance to various anti-pseudomonal compounds. The most potent combination is obviously that of a carbapenemase producing isolate usually enriched by resistance to quinolones and aminoglycosides leaving very limited options for antimicrobial treatment.

As far as newer carbapenem compounds are concerned, data suggest that doripenem does not offer advantages over other carbapenems against carbapenemase producing strains [126].

Tigecycline is an option for Gram-negative MDR pathogens but it cannot be used against *P. aeruginosa, Morganella morganii, Proteus* spp. and *Providencia* spp. because it is intrinsically vulnerable to their chromosomal-encoded efflux pumps [127].

Furthermore, time-kill studies on 12 MBL-producing *P. aeruginosa* isolates performed with aztreonam alone and in combination with ceftazidime and amikacin, showed bactericidal activity against one and eight isolates respectively. In the same study, colistin was bactericidal against all 12 isolates [128].

Category	Enzymatic family	Subfamily	Substrates	References
Acetyltransferases (AAC)	AAC(3)	I	Gentamicin	[11]
		II	Gentamicin Tobramycin	[48] [108,109]
		III	Gentamicin Tobramycin	
		IV	Gentamicin	
		VI	Gentamicin Tobramycin	
	AAC(6′)	I	Tobramycin Amikacin	[108,109]
		II	Tobramycin Gentamicin	
Nucleotidyltransferases (ANT)	ANT(2′)	I	Gentamicin Tobramycin	[109]
	ANT(4′)	IIa	Tobramycin Amikacin	[114,115]
		IIb	Tobramycin Amikacin	
	ANT(3′)		Streptomycin	[108]
Phosphoryltransferases (APH)	APH(3′)	II	Kanamycin Neomycin	[109] [116]
		IIb	Kanamycin	[117]
		IIb-like	Amikacin (weakly)	[113]
		VI	Amikacin Isepamicin	[110-112]
	APH(2′′)		Gentamicin Tobramycin	[110]

Table 6. Aminoglycoside-modifying enzymes found in *P. aeruginosa* isolates.

In fact, polymyxins and colistin in particular, are quite effective in the treatment of MDR *P. aeruginosa* infections [129,130]. The target of colistin is the bacterial cell membrane. More precisely, colistin interacts with the lipid A of lipopolysaccharides, allowing penetration through the outer membrane by displacing Ca^{2+} and Mg^{2+}. The insertion between the phospholipids leads to loss of membrane integrity and consequent bacterial cell death [131]. There are reports of resistance to polymyxin B [132-134] and colistin [135-137] in clinical isolates but they remain to date relatively rare for *P. aeruginosa* [24]. While in many cases the mechanism of clinical polymyxin resistance is unknown, substitution of the lipopolysaccharide lipid A with aminoarabinose has been shown to contribute to polymyxin resistance *in vitro* [138] and cystic fibrosis isolates [139]. Colistin is frequently associated with nephro- and neurotoxicity but both these adverse effects seem to be dose-dependent and reversible [140].

Another interesting option for the treatment of MDR *P. aeruginosa* is fosfomycin, an old antibacteial that has regained attention because of its *in vitro* activity against such isolates [140]. Fosfomycin inactivates the enzyme pyruvil-transferase, which is required for the synthesis of the cell wall peptidoglycan. In a review of the existing fosfomycin studies, 81.1% of 1529 patients were successfully treated for infections caused by *P. aeruginosa, Staphylococcus aureus, Staphylococcus epidermidis, Enterobacter* spp. and *Klebsiella* spp. Fosfomycin was administered together with aminoglycosides, cephalosporins and penicillines [141]. More studies are needed however to determine the future role of fosfomycin against MDR *P. aeruginosa* isolates.

6. Combination therapy

The application of combination therapy instead of monotherapy in cases of non-MDR *P. aeruginosa* remains to date a controversial issue [14]. Combination treatment against MDR strains instead seems to be some times necessary (for example in cases of pan-resistance or resistance to all except a single agent). In such cases better results are expected by the additive or subadditive activity of a combination or by the enhancement of a single active agent by an otherwise inactive drug [142].

Several old and newer studies have showed the increased activity *in vitro* of various antibiotic combinations against MDR *P. aeruginosa* (Table 7) even though, the mechanisms of positive interaction between the various agents are rarely known [142].

Antibiotic combination	References
Ticarcillin, Tobramycin, Rifampin	[143]
Cephalosporins, Quinolones	[144]
Ceftazidime, Colistin	[145]
Macrolides, Tobramycin, Trimethoprim, Rifampin	[146]
Polymyxin B, Rifampin	[147]
Polymyxin B, Imipenem	[148]
Colistin, Meropenem	[149]

Table 7. Enhanced activity of antibiotic combinations against MDR *P. aeruginosa*.

7. Conclusion

P. aeruginosa is a nosocomial pathogen of particular clinical concern not only because of its extraordinary resistance mechanisms armamentarium but also for its formidable ability to

http://dx.doi.org/10.5772/55616

adapt very well to the hospital environment. There are important challenges in the treatment of MDR *P. aeruginosa* strains and their isolation in healthcare settings poses serious infection control issues. For these reasons, the prudent use of antibiotics, mainly those used as last resort treatment like carbapenems is of outmost importance in order to prevent evolutionary pressure that may lead to the emergence of highly resistant clones.

Author details

Georgios Meletis[1,2] and Maria Bagkeri[3]

*Address all correspondence to: meletisg@hotmail.com

1 Aristotle University of Thessaloniki, School of Medicine,Thessaloniki, Greece

2 Department of Clinical Microbiology, Veroia General Hospital,Veroia, Greece

3 Department of Internal Medicine,Agios Dimitrios General Hospital of Thessaloniki, Greece

References

[1] Slama TG. Gram-negative antibiotic resistance: there is a price to pay. Crit Care 2008;12. (Sup4) S4.

[2] Kerr KG, Snelling AM. Pseudomonas aeruginosa: a formidable and ever-present adversary. J Hosp Infect 2009;73. 338–344.

[3] Mauldin PD, Salgado CD, Hansen IS, et al. Attributable hospital cost and length of stay associated with health care-associated infections caused by antibiotic-resistant Gram- negative bacteria. Antimicrob Agents Chemother 2010;54. 109–115.

[4] Tumbarello M, Repetto E, Trecarichi EM, et al. Multidrug- resistant Pseudomonas aeruginosa bloodstream infections: risk factors and mortality. Epidemiol Infect 2011;139. 1740-1749.

[5] Lambert PA. Mechanisms of antibiotic resistance in Pseudomonas aeruginosa. J R Soc Med 2002;95. 22-26.

[6] Moore NM, Flaws ML. Antimicrobial resistance mechanisms in Pseudomonas aeruginosa. Clin Lab Sci 2011; 24. 47-51.

[7] Hancock REW, & Brinkman F. Function of Pseudomonas porins in uptake and efílux. Annu Rev Microbiol 2002;56. 17-38.

[8] Tamber S, Ochs MM, Hancock REW. Role of the novel OprD family of porins in nutrient uptake in Pseudomonas aeruginosa. J Bacteriol 2006;188. 45-54.

[9] Lister PD, Wolter DJ, Hanson ND. Antibacterial-resistant Pseudomonas aeruginosa: Clinical impact and complex regulation of chromosomally encoded resistance mechanisms. Clin Micro Rev 2009;22. 582-610.

[10] Strateva T, Yordanov D. Pseudomonas aeruginosa – a phenomenon of bacterial resistance. J Med Microbiol 2009;58. 1133–1148.

[11] Schweizer HP. Efflux as a mechanism of resistance to antimicrobials in Pseudomonas aeruginosa and related bacteria: unanswered questions. Genet Mol Res 2003;2. 48-62.

[12] Girlich D, Naas T, Nordmann P. Biochemical characterization of the naturally occurring oxacillinase OXA-50 of Pseudomonas aeruginosa. Antimicrob Agents Chemother 2004;48.2043–2048.

[13] Kong KF, Jayawardena SR, Del Puerto A, et al. Characterization of poxB, a chromosomal-encoded Pseudomonas aeru-ginosa oxacillinase. Gene 2005;358. 82–92.

[14] Moore NM, Flaws ML. Treatment strategies and recommendations for Pseudomonas aeruginosa infections. Clin Lab Sci 2011;24. 52-56.

[15] Tipper DJ. Mode of action of beta-lactam antibiotics. Pharmacol Ther 1985;27.1-35.

[16] Hooper DC. Quinolone mode of action--new aspects. Drugs 1993;45. 8-14.

[17] Poole K. Efflux-mediated antimicrobial resistance. J Antimicrob Chemother 2005;56. 20–51.

[18] Kohler T, Van Delden C, Curty LK, et al. Overexpression of the MexEF-OprN multidrug efflux system affects cell-to-cell signaling in Pseudomonas aeruginosa. J Bacteriol 2001;183. 5213–5222.

[19] Westbrock-Wadman S, Sherman DR, Hickey MJ, et al. Characterization of a Pseudomonas aeruginosa efflux pump contributing to aminoglycoside impermeability. Antimicrob Agents Chemother 2004;43. 2975–2983.

[20] Pozzi G, Iannelli F, Oggioni MR, et al. Genetic elements carrying macrolide-efflux genes in streptococci. Curr. Drug Targets Infect Disord 2004; 4. 203–206.

[21] Li XZ, Poole K, Nikaido H. Contributions of MexAB-OprM and an ErmE homolog to intrinsic resistance of Pseudomonas aeruginosa to aminoglycosides and dyes. Antimicrob Agents Chemother, 2003;47. 27–33.

[22] Dozzo P, Moser, HE. New aminoglycoside antibiotics . Expert Opin Ther Pat 2010;20.1321-1341.

[23] Pagkalis S, Mantadakis E, Mavros MN, et al. Pharmacological considerations for the proper clinical use of aminoglycosides. Drugs 2011;71. 2277-2294.

[24] Poole K. Pseudomonas aeruginosa: resistance to the max. Front Microbiol 2011;2.65.

[25] Ambler RP. The structure of beta-lactamases. Philos Trans R Soc Lond B Biol Sci 1980;289. 321-331.

[26] Bush K, Jacoby GA, Medeiros AA. A functional classification scheme for beta-lactamases and its correlation with molecular structure. Antimicrob Agents Chemother 1995;39. 1211-1233.

[27] Falagas ME, Karageorgopoulos DEJ. Extended-spectrum beta-lactamase-producing organisms. J Hosp Infect 2009;73.345-354.

[28] Queenan AM, Bush K. Carbapenemases: the versatile beta-lactamases. Clin Microbiol 2007;20. 440-458.

[29] Arora S, Bal, M. AmpC β-lactamase producing bacterial iso-lates from Kolkata hospital. Indian J Med Res 2005;122. 224–233.

[30] Bratu S, Landman D, Gupta, J, et al. Role of AmpD, OprF and penicillin-binding proteins in β-lactam resistance in clinical isolates of Pseudomonas aeruginosa. J Med Microbiol 2007;56. 809–814.

[31] Reinhardt A, Kohler T, Wood P, et al. Development and persistence of antimicrobial resistance in Pseudomonas aeruginosa: a longitudinal observation in mechanically ventilated patients. Antimicrob Agents Chemother 2007;51. 1341–1350.

[32] Tam VH, Schilling AN, LaRocco MT, et al. Prevalence of AmpC over-expression in blood-stream isolates of Pseudomonas aeruginosa. Clin Microbiol Infect 2007;13, 413–418.

[33] Drissi M, Ahmed ZB, Dehecq B, et al. Antibiotic susceptibility and mechanisms of β-lactam resistance among clinical strains of Pseudomonas aeruginosa: first report in Algeria. Med Mal Infect 2008;38. 187-191.

[34] Vettoretti L, Floret N, Hocquet D, et al. Emergence of extensive-drug-resistant Pseudomonas aeruginosa in a French university hospital. Eur J Clin Microbiol Infect Dis 2009;28. 1217–1222.

[35] Upadhyay S, Sen MR, Bhattacharjee A. Presence of different β-lactamase classes among clinical isolates of Pseudomonas aeruginosa expressing AmpC β-lactamase enzyme. J Infect Dev Ctries 2010;4. 239–242.

[36] Xavier DE, Picao RC, Girardello R, et al. Efflux pumps expression and its association with porin down- regulation and β-lactamase production among Pseudomonas aeruginosa causing bloodstream infections in Brazil. BMC Microbiol 2010;10. 217.

[37] Dunne WM Jr, Hardin DJ.J. Use of several inducer and substrate antibiotic combinations in a disk approximation assay format to screen for AmpC induction in patient isolates of Pseudomonas aeruginosa, Enterobacter spp., Citrobacter spp., and Serratia spp. Clin Microbiol 2005;43. 5945-5949.

[38] Quale J, Bratu S, Gupta J, et al. Interplay of efflux system, ampC, and oprD expression in carbapenem resistance of Pseudomonas aeruginosa clinical isolates. Antimicrob Agents Chemother 2006;50. 1633-1641.

[39] Giedraitienė A, Vitkauskienė A, Naginienė R, et al. Antibiotic resistance mechanisms of clinically important bacteria. Medicina (Kaunas) 2011;47.137-146.

[40] Poirel L, Nordmann P. Acquired carbapenem-hydrolyzing β-lactamases and their genetic support. Curr Pharm Biotechnol 2002; 3. 117–127.

[41] Castanheira M, Toleman MA, Jones RN, et al. Molecular characterization of a β-lactamase gene, blaGIM-1, encoding a new subclass of metallo-β-lactamase. Antimicrob Agents Chemother 2004;48. 4654–4661.

[42] Walsh TR, Toleman MA, Poirel L, et al. Metallo-β-lactamases: the quiet before the storm? Clin Microbiol Rev 2005;18. 306–325.

[43] Naas T, Aubert D, Lambert T, et al. Complex genetic structures with repeated elements, a sul-type class 1 integron, and the blaVEB extended-spectrum β-lactamase gene. Antimicrob Agents Chemother 2006;50. 1745–1752.

[44] Bogaerts P, Bauraing C, Deplano A, et al. Emergence and dissemination of BEL- 1-producing Pseudomonas aeruginosa isolates in Belgium. Antimicrob Agents Chemother 2007;51. 1584–1585.

[45] Gupta V. Metallo β-lactamases in Pseudomonas aeruginosa and Acinetobacter species. Expert Opin Investig Drugs 2008;17. 131–143.

[46] Li H, Toleman MA, Bennett PM, et al. Complete Sequence of p07-406, a 24,179-base-pair plasmid harboring the blaVIM-7 metallo-β-lactamase gene in a Pseudomonas aeruginosa isolate from the United States. Antimicrob Agents Chemother 2008;52. 3099–3105.

[47] Castanheira M, Bell JM, Turnidge JD. Carbapenem resistance among Pseudomonas aeruginosa strains from India: evidence for nationwide endemicity of multiple metallo-β-lactamase clones (VIM-2, -5, -6, and -11 and the newly characterized VIM-18). Antimicrob Agents Chemother 2009;53. 1225–1227.

[48] Zhao WH, Chen G, Ito R, et al. Relevance of resistance levels to carbapenems and integron-borne blaIMP-1, blaIMP-7, blaIMP-10 and blaVIM-2 in clinical isolates of Pseudomonas aeruginosa. J Med Microbiol 2009;58. 1080–1085.

[49] Kotsakis SD, Papagiannitsis CC, Tzelepi E, et al. GES-13, a β-lactamase variant possessing Lys-104 and Asn-170 in Pseudomonas aeruginosa. Antimicrob Agents Chemother 2010;54. 1331–1333.

[50] Cambray G, Guerout AM, Mazel D. Integrons. Annu Rev Genet 2010;44. 141–166.

[51] Poirel L, Magalhaes M, Lopes M, et al. Molecular analysis of metallo-β-lactamase gene blaSPM-1-surrounding sequences from disseminated Pseudomonas aeruginosa isolates in Recife, Brazil. Antimicrob Agents Chemother 2004;48. 1406–1409.

[52] Picao RC, Poirel L, Gales AC, et al. Diversity of β-lactamases produced by ceftazidime-resistant Pseudomonas aeruginosa isolates causing bloodstream infections in Brazil. Antimicrob Agents Chemother 2009;53. 3908–3913.

[53] Picao RC, Poirel L, Gales AC, et al. Further identification of CTX-M-2 extended-spectrum β-lactamase in Pseudomonas aeruginosa. Antimicrob Agents Chemother 2009;53. 2225–2226.

[54] Paterson DL, Bonomo RA. Extendedspectrum β-lactamases: a clinical update. Clin Microbiol Rev 2005;18. 657–686.

[55] Lee K, Yum JH, Yong D, et al. Novel acquired metallo-β-lactamase gene, blaSIM-1, in a class 1 integron from Acinetobacter baumannii clinical isolates from Korea. Antimicrob Agents Chemother 2005;49. 4485–4491.

[56] Sacha P, Wieczorek P, Hauschild T, et al. Metallo-beta-lactamases of Pseudomonas aeruginosa--a novel mechanism of resistance to beta-lactam antibiotics. Folia Histochem Cytobiol 2008;46. 137-142.

[57] Pai H, Jacoby GA. Sequences of the NPS-1 and TLE-1 β-lactamase genes. Antimicrob Agents Chemother 2001;45. 2947–2948.

[58] Kalai BS, Achour W, Bejaoui M, et al. Detection of SHV-1 β-lactamase in Pseudomonas aeruginosa strains by genetic methods. Pathol Biol (Paris) 2009;57. e73–75.

[59] Celenza G, Pellegrini C, Caccamo M, et al. Spread of bla(CTX-M-type) and bla(PER-2) β-lactamase genes in clinical isolates from Bolivian hospitals. J Antimicrob Chemother 2006;57. 975–978.

[60] Jiang X, Zhang Z., Li, M, et al. Detection of extended-spectrum β-lactamases in clinical isolates of Pseudomonas aeruginosa. Antimicrob Agents Chemother 2006;50. 2990–2995.

[61] Rejiba S, Limam F, Belhadj C. Biochemical characterization of a novel extendedspectrum β-lactamase from Pseudomonas aeruginosa. Microb Drug Resist 2002;8. 9–13.

[62] al Naiemi N, Duim B, Bart, A. A CTX-M extended-spectrum β-lactamase in Pseudomonas aeruginosa and Stenotrophomonas maltophilia. J Med Microbiol 2006;55. 1607–1608.

[63] Sanschagrin F, Bejaoui N, Levesque RC. Structure of CARB-4 and AER-1 carbenicillin-hydrolyzing β-lactamases. Antimicrob Agents Chemother 42. 1998;1966–1972.

[64] Villegas MV, Lolans K, Correa A, et al. First identification of Pseudomonas aeruginosa isolates producing a KPC-type carbapenem-hydrolyzing β-lactamase. Antimicrob Agents Chemother 2007;51. 1553–1555.

[65] Wolter DJ, Khalaf N, Robledo IE, et al. Surveillance of carbapenem-resistant Pseudomonas aeruginosa isolates from Puerto Rican Medical Center Hospitals: dissemination of KPC and IMP-18 β-lactamases. Antimicrob Agents Chemother 2009;53. 1660–1664.

[66] Bert F, Vanjak D, Leflon-Guibout V, et al. IMP-4-producing Pseudomonas aeruginosa in a French patient repatriated from Malaysia: impact of early detection and control measures. Clin Infect Dis 2007;44. 764–765.

[67] Ryoo NH, Lee K, Lim JB, et al. Outbreak by meropenemresistant Pseudomonas aeruginosa producing IMP-6 metallo-β-lactamase in a Korean hospital. Diagn Microbiol Infect Dis 2009;63. 115–117.

[68] Iyobe S, Kusadokoro H, Takahashi A, et al. Detection of a variant metallo-β-lactamase, IMP-10, from two unrelated strains of Pseudomonas aeruginosa and an Alcaligenes xylosoxidans strain. Antimicrob Agents Chemother 2002;46. 2014–2016.

[69] Docquier JD, Riccio ML, Mugnaioli C, et al. IMP-12, a new plasmid-encoded metallo-β-lactamase from a Pseudomonas putida clinical isolate. Antimicrob Agents Chemother 2003;47. 1522–1528.

[70] Garza-Ramos U, Morfin-Otero R, Sader HS, et al. Metallo-β-lactamase gene bla(IMP-15) in a class 1 integron, In95, from Pseudomonas aeruginosa clinical isolates from a hospital in Mexico. Antimicrob Agents Chemother 2008;52. 2943–2946.

[71] Mendes RE, Toleman MA, Ribeiro J, et al. Integron carrying a novel metallo-β-lactamase gene, blaIMP-16, and a fused form of aminoglycoside-resistant gene aac(6′)-30/aac(6′)-Ib′: report from the SENTRY Antimicrobial Surveillance Program. Antimicrob Agents Chemother 2004;48. 4693–4702.

[72] Duljasz W, Gniadkowski M, Sitter S, et al. First organisms with acquired metallo-β-lactamases (IMP-13, IMP-22, and VIM-2) reported in Austria. Antimicrob Agents Chemother 2009;53. 2221–2222.

[73] Koh TH, Wang GC, Sng LH. IMP-1 and a novel metallo-β-lactamase, VIM-6, in fluorescent Pseudomonads isolated in Singapore. Antimicrob Agents Chemother 2004;48. 2334–2336.

[74] Siarkou VI, Vitti D, Protonotariou E, et al. Molecular epidemiology of outbreak-related Pseudomonas aeruginosa strains carrying the novel variant blaVIM-17 metallo-β-lactamase gene. Antimicrob Agents Chemother 2009;53. 1325–1330.

[75] Toleman MA, Simm AM, Murphy TA, et al. Molecular characterization of SPM-1, a novel metallo-β-lactamase isolated in Latin America: report from the SENTRY antimicrobial surveillance programme. J Antimicrob Chemother 2002;50. 673–679.

[76] Jovcic B, Lepsanovic Z, Suljagic V, et al. Emergence of NDM-1 Metallo-{beta}-Lactamase in Pseudomonas aeruginosa Clinical Isolates from Serbia. Antimicrob Agents Chemother 2011;55. 3929-3931.

[77] Rodriguez-Martinez JM, Poirel L, Nordmann P. Extended-spectrum cephalosporinases in Pseudomonas aeruginosa. Antimicrob Agents Chemother 2009;53. 1766–1771.

[78] Giuliani F, Docquier JD, Riccio ML, et al. OXA-46, a new class D β-lactamase of narrow substrate specificity encoded by a blaVIM-1-containing integron from a Pseudomonas aeruginosa clinical isolate. Antimicrob Agents Chemother 2005;49. 1973–1980.

[79] Juan C, Mulet X, Zamorano L, et al. Detection of the novel extended spectrum β-lactamase (ESBL) OXA-161 from a plasmid-located integron in Pseudomonas aeruginosa clinical isolates in Spain. Antimicrob Agents Chemother 2009;53. 5288–5290.

[80] Sevillano E, Gallego L, Garcia-Lobo JM. First detection of the OXA-40 carbapenemase in P. aeruginosa isolates, located on a plasmid also found in A. baumannii. Pathol Biol (Paris) 2009;57. 493–495.

[81] Watanabe M, Iyobe S, Inoue M, et al. Transferable imipenem resistance in Pseudomonas aeruginosa. Antimicrob Agents Chemother 1991;35.147–151.

[82] Lauretti L, Riccio ML, Mazzariol A, et al. Cloning and characterization of blaVIM, a new integron-borne metallo-β-lactamase gene from a Pseudomonas aeruginosa clinical isolate. Antimicrob Agents Chemother 1999;43. 1584–1590.

[83] Salabi AE, Toleman MA, Weeks J, et al. First report of the metallo-beta-lactamase SPM-1 in Europe. Antimicrob Agents Chemother 2010;54. 582.

[84] Yong D, Bell JM, Ritchie B, et al. A novel sub-group metallo-b-lactamase (MBL), AIM-1, emerges in Pseudomonas aeruginosa (PSA) from Australia. 47th Interscience Conference on Antimicrobial Agents and Chemotherapy. Chicago, IL, USA, 2007; Abstract C1–593.

[85] Poirel L, Weldhagen GF, Naas T, et al. GES-2, a class A beta-lactamase from Pseudomonas aeruginosa with increased hydrolysis of imipenem. Antimicrob Agents Chemother 2001;45. 2598-2603.

[86] Mavroidi A, Tzelepi E, Tsakris A, et al. An integron–associated β-lactamase (IBC-2) from Pseudomonas aeruginosa is a variant of the extended-spectrum β-lactamase IBC-1. J Antimicrob Chemother 2001;48. 627-630.

[87] El Garch F, Bogaerts P, Bebrone C, et al. OXA-198, an acquired carbapenem-hydrolyzing class D beta-lactamase from Pseudomonas aeruginosa. Antimicrob Agents Chemother 2011;55. 4828-4833.

[88] Poole K. Resistance to β-lactam antibiotics. Cell Mol Life Sci 2004;61. 2200–2223.

[89] Tomas M, Doumith M, Warner M, et al. Efflux pumps, OprD porin, AmpC β-lactamase, and multiresistance in Pseudomonas aeruginosa isolates from cystic fibrosis patients. Antimicrob Agents Chemother 2010;54. 2219–2224.

[90] Yoneda K, Chikumi H, Murata T, et al. Measurement of Pseudomonas aeruginosa multidrug efflux pumps by quantitative real-time polymerase chain reaction. FEMS Microbiol Lett 2005;243. 125-131.

[91] Farra A, Islam S, Strålfors A, et al. Role of outer membrane protein OprD and penicillin-binding proteins in resistance of Pseudomonas aeruginosa to imipenem and meropenem. Int J Antimicrob Agents 2008;31. 427-433.

[92] Gutiérrez O, Juan C, Cercenado E, et al. Molecular epidemiology and mechanisms of carbapenem resistance in Pseudomonas aeruginosa isolates from Spanish hospitals. Antimicrob Agents Chemother 2007;51. 4329-4335.

[93] Horii T, Muramatsu H, Morita M, et al. Characterization of Pseudomonas aeruginosa isolates from patients with urinary tract infections during antibiotic therapy. Microb Drug Resist 2003;9. 223-229.

[94] Wang J, Zhou JY, Qu TT, et al. Molecular epidemiology and mechanisms of carbapenem resistance in Pseudomonas aeruginosa isolates from Chinese hospitals. Int J Antimicrob Agents 2010;3. 486–491.

[95] Carmeli Y, Troillet N, Eliopoulos GM, et al. Emergence of antibiotic-resistant Pseudomonas aeruginosa: comparison of risks associated with different antipseudomonal agents. Antimicrob Agents Chemother 1999;43. 1379-1382.

[96] Jacoby GA. Mechanisms of resistance to quinolones. Clin Infect Dis 2005;41. 120–126.

[97] Drlica K, Hiasa H, Kerns R, et al. Quinolones: action and resistance updated. Curr Top Med Chem 2009;9. 981–998.

[98] Higgins PG, Fluit AC, Milatovic D, et al. Mutations in GyrA, ParC, MexR and NfxB in clinical isolates of Pseudomonas aeruginosa. Int J Antimicrob Agents 2003;21. 409–413.

[99] Henrichfreise B, Wiegand I, Pfister W, et al. Resistance mechanisms of multiresistant Pseudomonas aeruginosa strains from Germany and correlation with hypermutation. Antimicrob Agents Chemother 2007;51. 4062–4070.

[100] Rejiba S, Aubry A, Petitfrere S, et al. Contribution of parE mutation and efflux to ciprofloxacin resistance in Pseudomonas aeruginosa clinical isolates. J Chemother 2008;20. 749–752.

[101] Lee JK, Lee YS, Park YK, et al. Alterations in the GyrA and GyrB subunits of topoisomerase II and the ParC and ParE subunits of topoi-somerase IV in ciprofloxacin-resistant clinical isolates of Pseudomonas aeruginosa. Int J Antimicrob Agents 2005;25. 290–295.

[102] Muramatsu H, Horii T, Takeshita A, et al. Characterization of fluoroquinolone and carbapenem susceptibilities in clinical isolates of levofloxacin-resistant Pseudomonas aeruginosa. Chemotherapy 2005;51. 70–75.

[103] Nakano M, Deguchi T, Kawamura T, et al. Mutations in the gyrA and parC genes in fluoroquinolone-resistant clinical isolates of Pseudomonas aeruginosa. Antimicrob Agents Chemother 1997;41. 2289–2291.

[104] Schwartz T, Volkmann H, Kirchen S, et al. Real-time PCR detection of Pseudomonas aeruginosa in clinical and municipal wastewater and genotyping of the ciprofloxacin- resistant isolates. FEMS Microbiol Ecol 2006;57. 158–167.

[105] Poole K. Efflux-mediated resistance to fluoroquinolones in Gram-negative bacteria. Antimicrob Agents Chemother 2000;44. 2233–2241.

[106] Wolter DJ, Smith-Moland E, Goering RV, et al. Multidrug resistance associated with mexXY expression in clinical isolates of Pseudomonas aeruginosa from a Texas hospital. Diagn Microbiol Infect Dis 2004;50. 43–50.

[107] Zhanel GG, Hoban DJ, Schurek K, et al. Role of efflux mechanisms on fluoroquinolone resistance in Streptococcus pneumoniae and Pseudomonas aeruginosa. Int J Antimicrob Agents 2004;24. 529–535.

[108] Ramirez MS, Tolmasky ME. Aminoglycoside modifying enzymes. Drug Resist 2010;13. 151–171.

[109] Poole K. Aminoglycoside resistance in Pseudomonas aeruginosa. Antimicrob Agents Chemother 2005;49. 479–487.

[110] Kettner M, Milosovic P, Hletkova M, et al. Incidence and mechanisms of aminoglycoside resistance in Pseudomonas aeruginosa serotype O11 isolates. Infection 1995;23. 380–383.

[111] Kim JY, Park YJ, Kwon HJ, et al. Occurrence and mechanisms of ami-kacin resistance and its association with β-lactamases in Pseudomonas aeruginosa: a Korean nationwide study. J Antimicrob Chemother 2008;62. 479–483.

[112] Jin JS, Kwon KT, Moon DC, et al. Emergence of 16S rRNA methylase rmtA in colistin-only- sensitive Pseudomonas aeruginosa in South Korea. Int J Antimicrob Agents 2009;33. 490–491.

[113] Riccio ML, Pallecchi L, Fontana R, et al. In70 of plasmid pAX22, a blaVIM-1-containing integron carrying a new aminogly-coside phosphotransferase gene cas-sette. Antimicrob Agents Chemother 2001;45. 1249–1253.

[114] Shaw KJ, Munayyer H, Rather PN, et al. Nucleotide sequence analysis and DNA hybridization studies of the ant(4′)-IIa gene from Pseudomonas aeruginosa. Antimicrob Agents Chemother 1993;37. 708–714.

[115] Sabtcheva S, Galimand M, Gerbaud G, et al. Aminoglycoside resistance gene ant(4′)-IIb of Pseudomonas aeruginosa BM4492, a clinical isolate from Bulgaria. Antimicrob Agents Chemother 2003;47. 1584–1588.

[116] Miller GH, Sabatelli FJ, Naples L, et al. Resistance to aminoglycosides in Pseudomonas. Aminoglycoside Resistance Study Groups. Trends Microbiol 1994;2. 347–353.

[117] Hachler H, Santanam P, Kayser FH. Sequence and characterization of a novel chromosomal aminogly-coside phosphotransferase gene, aph (3′)-IIb, in Pseudomonas aeruginosa. Antimicrob Agents Chemother 1996;40. 1254–1256.

[118] Sobel ML, McKay GA, Poole K. Contribution of the MexXY multidrug transporter to aminogly-coside resistance in Pseudomonas aeruginosa clinical isolates. Antimicrob Agents Chemother 2003;47. 3202–3207.

[119] Hocquet D, Nordmann P, El Garch, et al. Involvement of the MexXY- OprM efflux system in emergence of cefepime resistance in clinical strains of Pseudomonas aeruginosa. Antimicrob Agents Chemother 2006;50. 1347–1351.

[120] Islam S, Oh H, Jalal S, et al. Chromosomal mechanisms of aminoglycoside resistance in Pseudomonas aeruginosa isolates from cystic fibrosis patients. Clin Microbiol Infect 2009;15. 60–66.

[121] Yamane K, Doi Y, Yokoyama K, et al. Genetic environments of the rmtA gene in Pseudomonas aeruginosa clinical isolates. Antimicrob Agents Chemother 2004;48. 2069–2074.

[122] Zhou Y, Yu H, Guo Q, et al. Distribution of 16S rRNA methylases among different species of Gram- negative bacilli with high-level resist-ance to aminoglycosides. Eur J Clin Microbiol Infect Dis 2010;29. 1349–1353.

[123] Gurung M, Moon DC, Tamang MD, et al. Emergence of 16S rRNA methylase gene armA and cocarriage of blaIMP-1 in Pseudomonas aeruginosa isolates from South Korea. Diagn Microbiol, Infect Dis 2010;68. 468–470.

[124] Doi Y, Ghilardi AC, Adams J, et al. High prevalence of metallo-β-lactamase and 16S rRNA methylase coproduction among imipenem- resistant Pseudomonas aeruginosa isolates in Brazil. Antimicrob Agents Chemother 2007;51. 3388–3390.

[125] Lincopan N, Neves P, Mamizuka EM, et al. Balanoposthitis caused by Pseudomonas aeruginosa co-producing metallo-β-lactamase and 16S rRNA methylase in children with hematological malignancies. Int J Infect Dis 2010;14. 344–347.

[126] Mushtaq S, Ge Y, Livermore DL. Comparative activities of doripenem versus isolates, mutants, and transconjugants of Enterobacteriaceae and Acinetobacter spp. with characterized b-lactamases. Antimicrob Agents Chemother 2004;48. 1113–1119.

[127] Dean CR, Visalli MA, Projan SJ, et al. Efflux-mediated resistance to tigecycline (GAR-936) in Pseudomonas aeruginosa PAO1. Antimicrob Agents Chemother 2003;47. 972-978.

[128] Oie S, Fukui Y, Yamamoto M, et al. In vitro antimicrobial effects of aztreonam, colistin, and the 3-drug combination of aztreonam, ceftazidime and amikacin on metallo b-lactamase-producing Pseudomonas aeruginosa. BMC Infect Dis 2009;9. 123.

[129] Montero M, Horcajada JP, Sorli L, et al. Effectiveness and safety of colistin for the treatment of multidrug-resistant Pseudomonas aeruginosa infections. Infection 2009;37. 461–465.

[130] Falagas ME, Rafailidis PI, Ioannidou E, et al. Colistin therapy for micro-biologically documented multidrug- resistant Gram-negative bacterial infections: a retrospective cohort study of 258 patients. Int J Antimicrob Agents 2010;35. 194–199.

[131] Giamarellou H. Treatment options for multidrug-resistant bacteria. Expert Rev Anti Infect Ther 2006;4. 601-618.

[132] Landman D, Bratu S, Alam M, et al. Citywide emergence of Pseudomonas aeruginosa strains with reduced susceptibility to poly-myxin B. J Antimicrob Chemother 2005;55. 954–957.

[133] Abraham N, Kwon DH. A single amino acid substitution in PmrB is associated with polymyxin B resistance in clinical isolate of Pseudomonas aeruginosa. FEMS Microbiol Lett 2009;298. 249–254.

[134] Barrow K, Kwon DH. Alterations in two-component regulatory systems of phoPQ and pmrAB are associated with polymyxin B resistance in clinical isolates of Pseudomonas aeruginosa. Antimicrob Agents Chemother 2009;53. 5150–5154.

[135] Johansen HK, Moskowitz SM, Ciofu O, et al. Spread of colistin resistant non- mucoid Pseudomonas aeruginosa among chronically infected Danish cystic fibrosis patients. J Cyst Fibros 2008;7. 391–397.

[136] Matthaiou DK, Michalopoulos A, Rafailidis PI, et al. Risk factors associated with the isolation of colistin-resistant Gram-negative bacteria: a matched case-control study. Crit Care Med 2008;36. 807–811.

[137] Samonis G, Matthaiou DK, Kofteridis D, et al. In vitro susceptibility to various antibiotics of colistin-resistant Gram-negative bacterial isolates in a general tertiary hospital in Crete, Greece. Clin Infect Dis 2010;5. 1689–1691.

[138] Moskowitz SM, Ernst RK, Miller SI. PmrAB, a two-component regulatory system of Pseudomonas aeruginosa that modulates resistance to cationic antimicrobial peptides and addition of aminoarabinose to lipid A. J Bacteriol 2004;186. 575–579.

[139] Ernst RK, Yi EC, Guo L, et al. Specific lipopolysaccha-ride found in cystic fibrosis airway Pseudomonas aeruginosa. Science 1999;286. 1561–1565.

[140] Giamarellou H, Poulakou G. Multidrug-resistant Gram-negative infections: what are the treatment options? Drugs 2009;69. 1879–1901.

[141] Falagas ME, Giannopoulou KP, Kokolakis GN, et al. Fosfomycin: use beyond urinary tract and gastrointestinal infections. Clin Infect Dis 2008;46. 1069-1077

[142] Rahal JJ. Novel antibiotic combinations against infections with almost completely resistant Pseudomonas aeruginosa and Acinetobacter species. Clin Infect Dis 2006; 43. Suppl 2:S95-99.

[143] Zuravleff JJ, Yu VL, Yee RB. Ticarcillin-tobramycin-rifampin: in vitro synergy of the triple combination against Pseudomonas aeruginosa. J Lab Clin Med 1983;101. 896–902.

[144] Fish DN, Choi MK, Jung R. Synergic activity of cephalosporins plus fluoroquinolones against Pseudomonas aeruginosa with resistance to one or both drugs. J Antimicrob Chemother 2002;50. 1045–1049.

[145] Gunderson BW, Ibrahim KH, Hovde LB, et al. Synergistic activity of colistin and ceftazidime against multiantibiotic-resistant Pseudomonas aeruginosa in an in vitro pharmacodynamic model. Antimicrob Agents Chemother 2003;47. 905–909.

[146] Saiman L, Chen Y, San Gabriel P, et al. Synergistic activities of macrolides antibiotics against Pseudomonas aeruginosa, Burkholderia cepacia, Stenotrophomonas maltophilia, and Alcaligines xylosoxidans isolated from patients with cystic fibrosis. Antimicrob Agents Chemother 2002;46. 1105–1107.

[147] Perez Urena MT, Barasoain I, Espinosa M, et al. Evaluation of different antibiotic actions combined with rifampicin. Chemotherapy 1975;27. 82–89.

[148] Chini NX, Scully B, DellaLatta P. Synergy of polymyxin B with imipenem and other antimicrobial agents against Acinetobacter, Klebsiella, and Pseudomonas species. Program and abstracts of the 38th Interscience Conference on Antimicrobial Agents and Chemotherapy (San Diego). Washington, DC: American Society for Microbiology 1998; Abstract E-56.

[149] Pankuch GA, Lin G, Seifect H, et al. Activity of meropenem with and without ciprofloxacin and colistin against Pseudomonas aeruginosa and Acinetobacter baumannii. Antimicrob Agents Chemother 2008;52. 333-336.

Chapter 3

Biofilms: A Challenge to Medical Fraternity in Infection Control

Silpi Basak, Monali N. Rajurkar, Ruchita O. Attal and Sanjay Kumar Mallick

Additional information is available at the end of the chapter

http://dx.doi.org/10.5772/55649

1. Introduction

Microbes have been characterized as planktonic, free-floating single cells. The morphological and physiological properties of microbes have been described as they grow in nutritionally rich culture media. Earlier very little thought have been given how microbes survive in the environment. But, the fact is, in natural environment, microbes are commonly found to be attached to surfaces as biofilms. Hence, the formation of surface attached microbial cells known as biofilms open a new horizon to study the micro-organisms.

Automatically, the question arises, "What is biofilm?" According to the recent definition, Biofilms can be defined as sessile communities of microbial cells irreversibly attached to a surface or interface or to each other which are embedded in a self produced matrix of extracellular polymeric biomolecules and are physiologically different from planktonic cells with respect to growth rate and gene transcription [1]. While studying Pseudomonas aeruginosa Davis and Geesay have shown that gene *alg*C controlling phosphomannomutase involved in alginate (exopolysacharide) synthesis is upregulated within 15 minutes of adhesion to a solid surface [2].

Biofilms are ubiquitous. They can be present on any surface – biotic or abiotic. Biofilms can be found on ship hulls, dairy and petroleum pipeline and rocks or pebbles at the bottom of streams or rivers. They can grow in hot acidic pools in Yellowstone National Park (USA) and on glaciers in Antarctica. Biofilms can form anywhere with easy access to water e.g. on tiles of floor, kitchen platform or clogged sink etc. They are also found on plants and can remain symbiotically or cause crop diseases like citrus canker, Pierce's disease of grapes etc [3]. Fossilised bioilms with 3.5 billion years are among the oldest records of life on earth [4]. Biofilms are also associated with biocorrosion of metals(microbiologically influenced corrosion.i.e.MIC) which affect kinetics of cathodic and or anodic reactions [5]. Biofilms can also grow in contact lenses, biomedical implants and transcutaneous devices.

Nearly every species of microorganisms e.g. bacteria, fungi, algae and protozoa have mechanisms to adhere to surfaces and to each other. It has been found that over 90% of all bacteria live in biofilms. Biofilms can be formed by single species of microorganism or by multiple species of bacteria, fungi, protozoa etc. Mixed species biofilms predominate in environment. Single species biofilm usually exist in a variety of infections and on medical implants and are the focus of current research [6].

Study of biofilm began when it was discovered that in natural aquatic system bacteria predominantly remain attached to surfaces [7]. The first recorded observation of biofilm was presented by Henrici in 1933 as 'it is quite evident that for the most part water bacteria are not free floating organisms, but grow upon submerged surfaces' [8]. The fouling of ship hulls by microbes in marine environment was already known to mankind. Hence, the study of biofilm has been started with marine bacteria, followed by fresh water microbial ecosystem and formation of biofilm on surface of eukaryotic tissue.

In early part of 20th Century it was difficult to observe biofilm as electron microscopy required complete dehydration of highly hydrated bioilm matrices and light microscopy was badly distorted by out-of-focus effects [1]. Though Confocal Laser Scanning Microscope (CLSM) was invented in 1950s it was never used to study bacteria. CLSM produces optical slices of complex structures, so out of focus effects are removed and it requires no sample preparations, so living microorganisms can be observed if fluorescent dye is introduced to observe the cells [1]. Hence, the modern biofilm era began with the use of Confocal Laser Scanning Microscope (CLSM) which showed the image of biofilm as sessile microbial cells embedded in matrix interspersed between open water channels [9].

The development of biofilm is a 5 stage process – 1) reversible attachment 2) irreversible attachment 3) early development 4) maturation 5) detachment or dispersal of cells. When the microbial cell reaches very closer to a surface (<1nm), the initial attachment depends upon the total attractive or repulsive forces between two surfaces. These forces include electrostatic and hydrophobic interactions, steric hindrance, van der Waals forces etc. Probably hydrophobic interactions play important role in primary adhesion [10]. The second stage of irreversible attachment employs molecular binding between specific adhesins and the surfaces [11].

The factors controlling biofilm formation are: i) recognition of attachment sites on a surface ii) nutritional cues iii) change of pH and temperature iv) exposure to antibiotics, chemical biocides, and host defense mechanisms e.g. complement system etc.

The gene expression in biofilm cells differ from planktonic cells and by 2D gel electrophoresis it had been found that in mature biofilm of *Pseudomonas aeruginosa* >300 proteins were detectable that were undetectable in planktonic cells [12].

During colonisation, microbial cells communicate via quorum sensing. In mature biofilm quorum sensing regulates formation of channels and pillar like structure for nutrient delivery.

Microbial cells in biofilms undergo cell density-dependent gene regulation i.e. quorum sensing and thus coordinate through signalling molecules called autoinducers. Autoinducers increase in concentration as a function of cell density [13]. Usually Gram positive bacteria use processed oligopeptides to communicate, where as Gram negative bacteria use N- acyl homoserine lactones (AHLs) as autoinducers [14]. The widespread AI-2 quorum-sensing system is found in several, Gram positive and Gram negative bacteria also [15]. For acyl-HSL quorum-sensing, an enzyme belong to Lux I family is required for synthesis of signal from cellular metabolites [16]. For AI-2 quorum-sensing system which has been implicated in interspecies communication, the synthesis of signalling molecule is directed by the Lux S gene product [17]. The ahyR/ I acyl- HSL quorum sensing system of Aeromonas hydrophila has been shown to be required for biofilm maturation [12]. Similarly the Lux S type quorum sensing system in *Streptococcus mutants* is also involved in biofilm development. Lux S system of *Salmonella* enterica serovar Typhimurium is required for biofilm formation on human gallstones [18].

Duenne described biofilm architecture as underwater coral reef with pyramid or mushroom shaped projections from the surface and channels and caverns running through out [19]. Using CLSM, Lawrence et al has shown that Pseudomonas biofilms were more tightly packed at the surface and less dense near the periphery whereas *Vibrio parahaemolyticus* biofilms show greatest cell density near the periphery [20].

The adherent cells in a biofilm are embedded with a self produced matrix of extracellular polymeric biomolecules. 97% of a biofilm matrix is water. A complex of secreted polymers, absorbed nutrients and metabolites, cell lysis product and even particulate materials from the surrounding environment can form matrix. Actually the matrix surrounds, anchors and protects surface-bound microbes. The matrix actually prevent the access of antimicrobials and disinfectants and confer protection against environmental stresses such as UV radiation, pH shifts, osmotic shock and dessication [21].

Besides microbial cells all major classes of macromolecules i.e. proteins, polysaccharides, nucleic acids can be observed within a biofilm. Even transformation, transduction and conjugation result in gene transfer amongst the cells in biofilm.

Biofilms are formed by many bacterial species of medical importance e.g. *Staphylococcus epidermidis, Staphylococcus aureus, Enterococci, Streptococcus mutans, Pseudomonas aeruginosa, E.coli* O157:H7, *Neisseria gonorrhoeae, Vibrio cholerae, Nontuberculous mycobacteria* (NTM) etc [6]. Amongst fungi - Candida albicans can usually form biofilm [22]. The two most intensely studied biofilms are produced by: *Staphylococcus epidermidis* and *Pseudomonas aeruginosa.*

1.1. Biofilms and human disease

The microbial biofilm has received much attention recently because biofilm mode of growth may be the key factor in persistent or chronic infections. The biofilms can act as nidus of acute infections and the microbial cells from biofilm are released at any one time during chronic infection [23]. Clinicians are very much concerned about the fact that it is really difficult to eradicate biofilm bacteria with antibiotics. Even in immunocompetent host the biofilm growth are rarely resolved by host's immune system as antigen may be hidden and key ligands may be repressed [24]. Biofilms are associated with kidney stones of infective origin, formation of dental plaques, infections in cystic fibrosis, infections of permanent indwelling devices such as joint prosthesis & heart valves, intrauterine devices (IUDs) and urinary catheters etc [25].

However in many chronic infections both the biofilm and planktonic growth may coexist. Parsek and Singh in 2003 have proposed few criteria to define the role of biofilms in human diseases [12]: a) the causative bacteria are surface associated b) examination of infected tissue shows bacteria living in microcolonies and embedded in extracellular matrix c) infection is usually confined to a particular site and dissemination occurs as a secondary phenomenon d) the infection is difficult to eradicate with antibiotics though the causative bacteria are susceptible to that antibiotics in planktonic state.

1.1.1. Infection-related kidney stones

15-20% of kidney stones occur in the setting of urinary tract infections. Infact, infection stones are produced by interplay between infecting bacteria and mineral substrates derived from urine resulting in formation of a complex biofilm. Microscopic analysis of stone has revealed that bacteria are organized in microcolonies and surrounded by an anionic matrix composed of both polysaccharides and crystallized minerals [26]. It requires an alkaline environment to decrease solubility of phosphate, increased concentration of NH_4^+ for struvite and CO_3^- for carbon apatite formation as these are major constituents of this type of stone. The normal urine is not saturated with struvite and carbon apatite. The alkaline pH of urine occurs in infection with urease producing organisms like *Proteus, Providencia, Klebsiella* and *Pseudomonas* species. It is hypothesized that biofilms provide localized and concentrated urease activity to form stones [26].

1.1.2. Bacterial endocarditis

The primary lesion in endocarditis is due to vegetation (valve biofilm), which is composed mainly of bacteria and their products, platelets and fibrin derived from circulation with the damaged endothelial surface as substratum. Durack in1975, developed nonbacterial thrombotic endocarditis by leaving a polyethylene catheter in contact with aortic valve of a rabbit and showed how bacterial microcolonies were formed within 24 hours [27].

1.1.3. Airway infections in cystic fibrosis

Cystic fibrosis (CF), a common inherited disease of lower respiratory tract is caused by mutation in the gene which encodes Cystic fibrosis transmembrane regulator protein (CFTR). CFTR functions as a chloride ion channel protein [1]. Chloride ion transport is severely impaired when CFTR is defective in CF patients, resulting in hyperviscous mucus. Initially CF patients suffer from intermittent respiratory infections but in late stage permanent infection with *P. aeruginosa* occurs. It has been found that even with higher antibiotics given parenterally *P. aeruginosa* could not be eradicated from sputum of CF patients in the late stage and it may persist for the rest of the patient's life. In permanent infection phase of CF patients, *P. aeruginosa* biofilm may be found in airways. Another interesting finding is emergence of *P. aeruginosa* with mucoid phenotype in late stage CF patients [28]. This mucoid material is a polysaccharide i.e. alginate which probably prevent antibody coating and opsonic phagocytosis. In fact, biofilm protects *P. aeruginosa* from antimicrobials and host defenses. Genetic fingerprinting studies show same strain of *P. aeruginosa* can persist in CF patients for decades leading to chronic inflammation and decline in lung function and ultimately respiratory failure [29].

1.1.4. Endodontics

Biofilms also play a major role in causing dental caries, gingivitis, periodontitis, apical periodontitis etc [30].The anatomical complexities in root canal system provide favourable condition for biofilm formation, which is actually initiated by invasion of pulp chamber by oral flora after tissue breakdown. Facultative or strict anaerobes are more frequently associated than aerobic microorganisms. *Porphyromonas gingivalis* is the primary agent responsible for periodontitis [31]. Endodontic biofilm can be—i) intracanal, ii) extraradicular, iii) periapical and iv) foreign body centered. Foreign body centered biofilm is a major complication associated with prosthesis and implant supported prosthesis [32].

1.1.5. other conditions

Similarly during acute phase of osteomyelitis, microscopical examination have shown biofilm formation on infected bone surfaces [33]. In chronic prostatitis, adherent bacterial colonies on the surface of prostatic duct have been observed on microscopical studies, even in culture negative cases [34].

1.1.6. Indwelling medical devices

Biofilms can develop on indwelling medical devices like prosthetic heart valve, pacemakers, central venous catheter, urinary catheter, contact lenses, intrauterine devices etc. and can cause persistent infections which are usually lethal. Scanning electron microscopy clearly shows biofilm formation at the tip of urinary catheter kept for 7 days. On medical devices, biofilms are most commonly formed by coagulase negative Staphylococci (CoNS) especially *S. epidermidis* followed by *S. aureus, Enterococci, Pseudomonas aeruginosa* etc.

Biofilms can develop on both types of contact lenses i.e. soft and hard and also on contact lens storage cases. *Pseudomonas aeruginosa, Staphylococcus aureus, Staphylococcus epidermidis, E.coli,* Candida species can adhere to contact lenses [35]. Evidence of biofilm on contact lenses and it's storage cases have been reported from patients with microbial kerattis [36]. The rate of prosthetic valve endocarditis (PVE) range from 0.5% to 4% [37]. Coagulase negative Staphylococci are the commonest early colonizers after surgical implantation of prosthetic valve whereas *Streptococcus viridans* most commonly colonize during late PVE (i.e. 12 months following valve replacement) [38]. Though *S. aureus,* Gram negative coccobacilli or fungi may also be responsible for PVE.

Infection with central venous catheter is a quite common device related infection. Biofilms have been shown by CLSM to be present outside the catheter or inner lumen [34].

In S. epidermidis biofilm initial adherence is by polysaccharide adhesin (PSA) and accumulation of cells is due to production of polysaccharide intercellular adhesin (PIA).) PIA is encoded by *ica* (intercellular adhesin) operon *ica* ADBC [39]. The *icaR* gene regulates *ica* operon. Production of PIA is also subject to ON - OFF switching (phase variation). Majority of clinical isolates of *S. aureus* also possess *ica* structural genes [40].

1.1.7. Health care Associated Infections (HAI) and biofilm

Catheter Associated Urinary Tract Infection(CA-UTI) is the commonest (>40%) HAI [41]. Nosocomial bacteriuria or candiduria develops in 25% of patients having urinary catheter for >7 days with a daily risk of 5% [42]. Most infected urinary catheters are covered by a thick biofilm containing infecting microorganisms. A biofilm forms intraluminally or extraluminally or both ways.

With the increasing use of vascular access devices, catheter related bloodstream infection (CR-BSI), septic thrombophlebitis, endocarditis and other metastatic infections e.g.lung abscess osteomyelitis and endophthalmitis etc. are also increasing. In the United States out of 5 million Central Venous cathetes used each year, 3-8% lead to BSI [43]. The initiation of catheter colonization occurs with the formation of a biofilm in the catheter lumen. Moreove the resistance levels of biofilm associated organisms may be much higher than those of planktonic organisms [44]. After stoppage of antimicrobial therapy, the biofilm associated organisms resurge and cause another clinical infectios. A recent approach to reduce CR-BSI is bundles of preventive measures, which means a group of preventive measures, when executed together, result in better outcomes than when implemented alone [45]. This included handwashing, using full barrier precautions during insertion of central venous line, cleaning the skin with chlorhexidine. The femoral site should be avoided if possible and catheters should be removed as early as possible.

Hospital acquired pnumoniais are the second most common cause of HAI and has the highest morbidity and mortality of all HAIs [46]. The initial step in pathogenesis of HAP is colonization of patient's oropharynx with resistant hospital pathogen. The endotracheal tube lumen is a nidus for the growth of bacteria within the biofilm. Hand washing and Personal protective equipment (PPE) must be used to reduce the incidence of HAP/ Ventilator assaociated pneumonia (VAP).

1.1.8. Resistance of biofilm to antimicrobials and disinfectants

It has been observed that biofilms are not easily eradicated even by cidal antimicrobials, quarternary ammonium compounds, halogens and halogen release agents. The crux of the problem is the presence of persisters within the biofilms that can rebound when antibiotic concentration falls. The causes are multifactorial – i) restricted penetration of antimicrobials within the biofilm architecture, ii) decreased growth rate of bacterial cells forming the biofilm, iii) expression of resistance gene by the bacterial cells within the biofilm etc [47]. Restricted penetration of antimicrobials may occur as negatively charged exopolysaccharide restrict permeation of positively charged antibiotics e.g. Aminoglycoside and exopolymer matrix also restrict diffusion of antimicrobial within the biofilm. Synergy between retarded diffusion and degradation by enzymes (e.g. β-lactamase) also provide effective resistance to antimicrobials. Fluoroquinolones are very effective in stopping the growth of a biofilm but restricted diffusion can protect the microbial cells within the biofilm [48]. All antimicrobials are more effective in killing rapidly growing cells. Penicillin & ampicillin do not kill non-growing cells as rate of killing is directly proportional to rate of growth for these two antibiotics. Even cephalosporins, aminoglycosides & fluroquinolones can kill rapidly dividing cells more effectively. Multiple drug resistance (MDR) pumps may play a role in biofilm resistance at low antibiotic concentration. Sometimes unknown MDR pumps might be over expressed in biofilm e.g. for chloramphenicol in *E. coli* biofilm. Moreover, the biofilms increase the opportunity of gene transfer beteen the microorganisms and can convert a previously avirulent commensal organism to a highly virulent pathogen. The enhanced efficiency of gene transfer in biofilms also fascilitates the spread of antibiotic resistance and virulence factors [49]. Though most of the research works deals with single species biofilms, multispecies biofilm amongst different bacteria and interkingdom biofilms between fungus Candida albicans and various bacterial species are also gaining importance in causing different diseases [50]. Biofilm formation is a major virulence factor for Candida albicans and Candida biofilms are difficult to eradicate due to their high resistance to antifungals. A recent study has reported that within the biofilm Staphylococcus aureus was attached uniquely with the pseudohyphae of Candida albicans. This synergistic interaction resulted in differential protein expressions which are actually virulence factors for Staphylcoccus aureus. This indicate C. albicans may enhance S.aureus pathogenesis [51]. Recently it has been reported that co-existence of S.aureus and C.albicans in a biofilm resulted in increased Vancomycin resistance in S.aureus [52] However antagonistic interaction has been reported between *Pseudomonas aeruginosa and Candida albicans* [53].

It is not possible to detect the antimicrobial resistance of biofilms by conventional methods of disc diffusion and broth microdilution as per CLSI guideline because these methods are only meant for planktonic cells.

1.1.9. Biofilms and altruism

Biofilms are like small cities and encourage altruism. Microbial cells within biofilm often sacrifice their maximum growth rate to use the available community resources more efficiently. In a biofilm atleast some of the microbial cells experience nutrient limitation and exist in a slow growing state [54]. In this process while individual cells are disadvantaged, the microbial community as a whole is benefited. Hence, it is said that biofilms are the colonial way of life of microorganisms.

Detection of biofilms can be done by both phenotypic methods and genotypic methods. In phenotypic methods biofilms are detected by Congo red agar method(CRA),Plastic tube method(TM), Tissue culture plate method(TCP) and Confocal Laser Scanning Microscopy (CLSM). In genotypic method, usually Polymerase chain reaction (PCR) for amplification of microbial DNA, coding for biofilm formation is done. The phenotypic methods are easy and cheap compared to genotypic method.

Hence, the present study was undertaken to detect the biofilm producing organisms, isolated from different clinical specimens in our laboratory.

2. Material and methods

The present study was conducted from 2009 to 2012. A total number of 350 bacterial and 50 Candida strains were studied. The microbial strains were isolated from different clinical specimens like urine, blood, pus and wound swab, endotracheal aspirate, urinary catheter tip, central venous catheter tip etc. All the microbial strains were identified by conventional methods [55]. We used microtitre plate biofilm assay to detect microbial attachment to an abiotic surface [56].

Steps:

1. The microbial cells were grown in Brain heart infusion broth overnight.
2. On next day, the cultures were diluted 1:100 using the brain heart infusion broth.
3. 100μl of each diluted culture was inoculated into each of three wells in a microtiter plate which has not been tissue culture treated. The plates were covered by the lid and was incubated at optimal growth temperature [56] for 48 hours
4. Then the wells were washed twice to remove planktonic cells.
5. Microbial cells which were adhered to the wells were subsequently stained with crystal violet solution that allowed visulisation of the attachment pattern. 125 μl of 0.1% crystal violet solution was added to each well and stained for 10 minutes at room temperature.
6. The microtiter plates were shaken and the crystal violet solution was removed.
7. The plates were washed successively twice with distilled water. Any crystal violet that is not specifically staining the adherent microbial cells were removed by this washing step.
8. The microtiter plates were then inverted and tapped vigorously on tissue paper to remove any excess liquid.
9. The microtiter plates were then air dried. The dried microtiter plates may be stored at room temperature for several weeks.
10. This surface associated dye was solubilized by adding ethanol or any other solvent for semiquantitative assessment of biofim formed. 200μl of 95% ethanol or other appropriate solvent [56] was then added to each stained well and was kept for 10 to 15 minutes
11. The contents of each well were mixed by pipetting and then 125μl of the crystal violet / ethanol solution from each well was transferred to a separate well of another 96 well microtiter plate maintaining the same sequence.

12. Then the optical density of each well containing 125μl solution was measured at a wavelength of 545nm in an ELISA reader. As each strain was put in triplicate the average of the three readings were taken.

The biofilm formation of different strains were classified in three groups according to the cut off OD. The cut off OD (ODc) for the microtiter plate test was defined as three standard deviations above the mean OD of the negative control. Isolates were classified into four groups as nonadheremt, weakly adherent, moderately adherent and strongly adherent according to Stepanovi et al [57].

3. Observation and results

Out of 350 bacterial strains studied, 90 were *Pseudomonas aeuginosa*, 80 were *E. coli*, 35 were *Klebsiella pneumoniae*, 80 were *Coagulase positive Staphylococci*, 30 were Coagulase negative 35 included Proteus sp(5), *Vibrio cholerae*(3), *Acinetobacter baumanii*(4), Enterococcus sp.(23). Out of 50 Candida strains 23 were *Candida albicans*, 16 were *Candida tropicalis*, 2 were *Candida dubliensis*, 6 were *Candida krusei* and 3 were *Candida glabrata*. Amongst 350 bacterial strains, 153(43.7%) and out of 50 *Candida* species 28(56%) were biofilm producers respectively. Amongst 50 Candida species, 11 (22%) were strong biofilm producers, and 6/11 (54.5%) were *Candida albicans*.

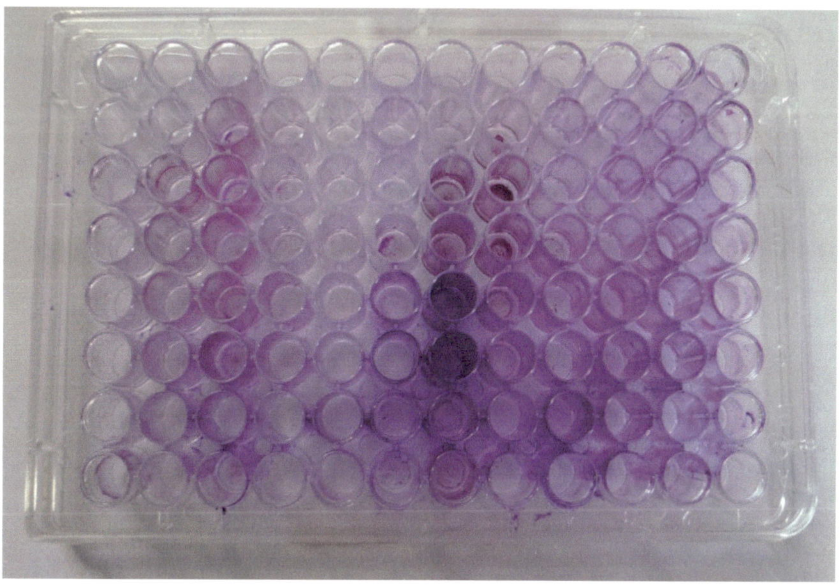

Figure 1. Microtitre plate biofilm assay for detection of microbial attachment

Maximum 65(72.2%) of *Pseudomonas aeruginosa* strains produced biofilms. 51(33.3%) biofilm producing bacterial strains were isolated from catheterized urine samples or patients having other medical devices. 108(70.6%) bacterial strains producing biofilms were isolated from patients having chronic infections eg persistent or recurrent UTI, Chronic obstructive airway disease, cystic fibrosis etc.

In our study the cut off OD(ODc) was 0.003. The biofilm forming organisms are grouped into weak group (OD ≥ 0.003 to 0.006), moderate group (OD ≥ 0.006 to 0.012) and strong group (OD > 0.012).

	Newer β – lactamases producers							Non β – lactamase producers
Organisms	**ESBL Only**	**AmpC Only**	**MBL Only**	**ESBL + AmpC**	**ESBL + MBL**	**AmpC + MBL**	**ESBL + AmpC +MBL**	
P.aeruginosa [90]	10	14	10	23	-	-	-	33
Strongly adherent biofilm producing P.aeruginosa	7	6	4	11	-	-	-	5
E.coli [80]	10	7	4	38	1	-	1	19
Strongly adherent biofilm producing E.coli	6	4	2	20	1	-	-	1
Klebsiella pneumonia [35]	3	2	1	8	2	-	-	19
Strongly adherent biofilm producing K. pneumoniae	1	1	1	4	1	-	-	2
Proteus species [5]	3	1	-	1	-	-	-	-
Strongly adherent biofilm producing Proteus species	1	-	-	-	-	-	-	-
Acinetobacter baumani [4]	1	1	2	-	-	-	-	-
Strongly adherent biofilm producing Acinetobacter baumani	-	-	2	-	-	-	-	-

Table 1. Incidence of strong biofilm producers amongst newer β – lactamases producing strains

It was observed that out of 57 newer β – lactamases (Extended spectrum β – lactamases i.e. ESBL, Amp C β – lactamases and Metallobetalactamases i.e. MBL only and in combination)

producing Pseudomonas aeruginosa 28 (49.1%) were strongly adherent biofilm producers, compared to only 5/33 (15.1%) non β – lactamase producers. Amongst the 120 Enterobacteriaceae strains studied. 82 (68.3%) were newer β – lactamases producers, whereas 48/82 (58.5%) were strong biofilm producers and only 3/38 (7.9%) non β – lactamase producing strains were strong biofilm producers.

Organisms	Methicillin resistant	Methicillin sensitive
Coagulase positive Staphylococcus [80]	34	46
Strongly adherent biofilm producing Coagulase positive Staphylococcus	14	2
Coagulase negative Staphylococci (CONS) [30]	11	19
Strongly adherent biofilm producing Coagulase negative Staphylococci (CONS)	4	2

Table 2. Incidence of strong biofilm producing Methicillin resistant Staphylococcus strains.

Table 2 shows amongst the Methicillin Resistant Staphylococcus aureus (MRSA) strains, 14/34 (41.2%) and Methicillin Resistant Coagulase negative Staphylococci (MR – CONS) 4/11 (36.4%) were strong biofilm producers compared to 2/46 (4.3%) *Methicillin sensitive Staphylococcus aureus* (MSSA) and 2/19 (10.5%) Methicillin sensitive CONS.

Out of 23 Enterococcus species 13/23 (56.5%)were High level Aminoglycoside Resistant (HLAR) strains and it was also found that 8/13 (61.5%) HLAR strains were strong biofilm producers compared to only 2/10 (20%) of non HLAR strains.

4. Discussion

Our Hospital is a tertiary care centre in a rural setup. Though CLSM is the best phenotypic method, it could not be used as it is very costly. We did a pilot study with Staphylococci in 2008 and found 33% of Staphylococcus aureus and 44.7% of Coagulase Negative Staphylococci (CONS) were biofilm producers and amongst the 3 phenotypic methods tissue culture plate method gave the best results [58]. The present study correlated well with reports of other authors that Extended Spectrum β-Lactamase (ESBL) producing strains, Methicillin Resistant Staphylococcs aureus(MRSA) were more adherent to microtitre plate than Non ESBL and Non MRSA strains (Figure 2).

Lee et al in 2008 have also reported a positive correlation between biofilm formation and ESBL producing Acinetobacter baumanii [59]. Norouzi et al in 2010 have reported that in their study 14% ESBL producing Pseudomonas aeruginosa has formed strongly adherent biofilm compared to only 4% of non-ESBL producing Pseudomonas aeruginosa [60]. It has also been

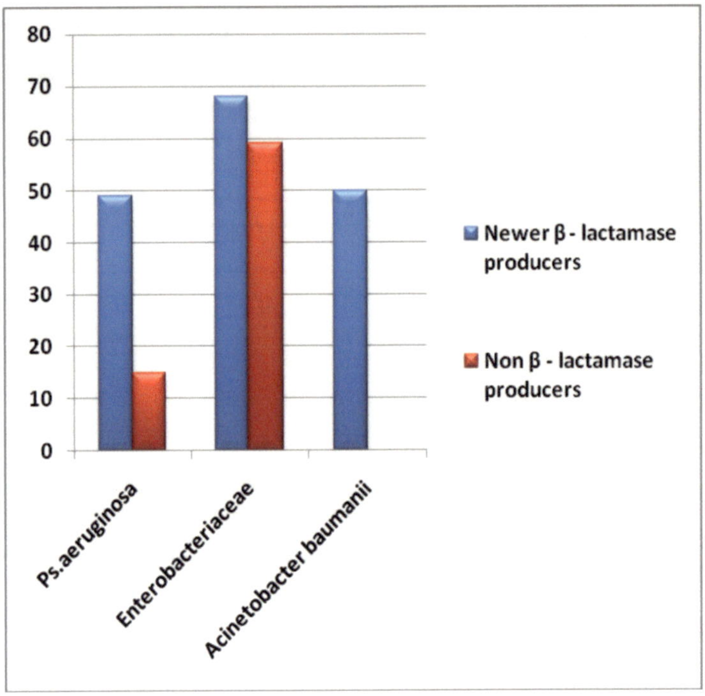

Figure 2. Strogly adherent biofilm producing strains (%) amongst newer β – lactamase producers and non β – lactamase producers

reported that, biofilm production was higher amongst MRSA strains as compared to Metthicillin sensitive S.aureus (MSSA) strains [61].

5. Treatment and control strategies

As far as the treatment of the persistant infection with medical device is concerned, the first step is to remove the infected indwelling medical device. Several control strategies have been proposed for biofilms e.g. systemic ciprofloxacin therapy in catheterized patients [1], latex catheter coated with silicone or silver hydrogel, catheter containing or use of antibiotics specially combination of Rifampicin and Minocyclin into material of indwelling catheters [62], Nitrofurazon coating, pretreatment of catheter surfaces with Furanones or Liposomes, Targetting the irradication of extra cellular polymeric biomolecules by enzymes [63] etc. Other strategies include disinfection of the insertion sites [64], surgical site irrigation, with biocides or antimicrobial locks to reduce indwelling catheter associated infections [65]. Cartin and Donlan have reported the ability of bacteriophage to degrade biofilm formation by Staphylococcus epidermidis [66]. Vejborg and Klemn have reported blocking of bacterial biofilm formation by a fish protein coating [67]. In dentistry, other than sodium hypochlorite irrigation, the newer techniques for biofilm eradication include ultrasonic irrigation, Ozone, plasma dental probe, photoactive disinfection with low energy LASER etc [32].

To prevent biofilm formation, the physical approaches like the use of low strength electrical field [68], electromagnetic field or ultrasound along with antibiotic therapy [69] are also very promising. A novel treatment based on disruption of quorum sensing system to inhibit biofilm formation has also been suggested by many workers [70]. Even the workers have suggested the inhibition of transcription of genes that are activated or repressed during initial biofilm formation will also help to prevent persistent infection due to biofilms. All these control strategies are on experimental basis and are not applicable for medical devices and have their own limitations to be used cuurently in patients.

To conclude, we must say biofilm develops slowly but has a major impact both clinically and economically on overall outcome of the patients treatment. The authors feel that, EARLY DETECTION AND NEWER TREATMENT OPTIONS FOR BIOFILM ASSOCIATED INFECTIONS ARE NEED OF THE HOUR.

Author details

Silpi Basak*, Monali N. Rajurkar, Ruchita O. Attal and Sanjay Kumar Mallick

Department of Microbiology, Jawaharlal Nehru Medical College, Wardha (M.S.), India

References

[1] Doulam RM, Costerton JW. Biofilms: Survival mechanisms of clinically relevant micro-organisms. Clin Microbiol Rev. 2002; 15(2): 167-193.

[2] Davis DG, Geesy GG. Regulation of the alginate biosynthesis gene algC in Pseudomonas aeruginosa during biofilm development in continuous culture. Appl Environ Microbiol. 1995; 61: 860-7.

[3] Introduction to Biofilms: Negative and positive impacts of biofilm. Available from: http://www.cs.montana.edu/ross/personal/intro-biofilms-s3.html.

[4] Schopf JW, Hayes JM, Walter MR. Evolution on earth's earliest ecosystems: recent progress and unsolved problems. In: Schopf JW Ed, Earth's earliest biosphere. Princeton University Press, New Jersy, 1983; 15:143-147.

[5] Jones DA, Amy PS. A thermodynamic interpretation of microbiologically influenced corrosion. Corros2002;58:638-645.

[6] Toole GO, Kaplan HB, kolter R. Biofilm formation as microbial development. Annu Rev Microbiol.2000; 54:49-79.

[7] Geesy GG, Richardson WT, Yeomans HG, Irvin RT, Costeton JW. Microscopic examination of natural sessile bacterial populations from an alpine stream. Can.J.Microbiol. 1977;23(12): 1733-1736.

[8] Henrici AT. Studies of fresh water bacteria. Adirect microscopic technique. J.Bacteriol. 1933;25: 277-287.

[9] Stoodley P, Sauer K, Davies D G, Costerton J W. Biofilms as complex differentiated communities. Annu Rev Microbiol. 2002; 56: 187: 209.

[10] Carpentier B, Cerf O. Biofilms and their consequences, with particular reference to hygiene in food industry. J Appl Bacteriol. 1993; 75: 499-511.

[11] An. YH, Dickinson RB and Doyle RJ. Mechanism of bacterial adhesion and pathogenesis of implant and tissue infections, In: Anand YH and Fridman RJ editors. Handbook of bacterial adhesions: Principles, methods and applications. Humana press; Totowa. NJ: 2000. P: 1-27.

[12] Sauer K, Camper AK, Ehrlich GD, Costerton JW, Davies DG. Pseudomonas aeruginosa displays multiple phenotypes during development as a biofilm. J Bacteriol 2002; 184: 1140-54.

[13] Miller MB, Bassler BL. Quorum sensing in bacteria. Ann. Rev. Microbiol. 2001;55:165-199.

[14] Miller MB, Bassler BL. Quorum sensing in bacteria. Annu Rev Microbiol 2001; 55: 165-99.

[15] Bassler B L, Small talk. Cell-to-cell communication in bacteria. Cell 2002; 109: 421-4.

[16] Schafer AL. Generation of Cell-to-cell signals in quorum sensing: acyl homo serine lactone synthase activity of a purified Vibrio fischeri Lux I protein. Proc Natl Acad Sci. USA 1996; 93: 9505-9.

[17] Schauder S, Shokat K, Surette MG, Bassler BL. The Lux S family of bacterial autoinducers: biosynthesis of a novel quorum-sensing signal molecule. Mol Microbiol 2001; 41: 463-76.

[18] Prouty AM. Biofilm formation and interaction with the surfaces of gallstones by Salmonella spp. Infect Immun 2002; 70: 2640-9.

[19] Dunne WH Jr. Bacterial adhesion: seen any good biofilm lately. Clin Microbiol Rev. 2002 Apr: 155-166.

[20] Lawrence JR, Korber DR, Hoyle BD, Costerton JW, Caldwell DE. Optical sectioning of microbial biofilms. J Bacteriol. 1991: 173:6558-67.

[21] Flemming HC. Bifilms and environmental protection. Water Sci Technol. 1993; 27:1-10.

[22] Baillie GS, Douglas LJ. Role of dimorphism in the development of Candida albicans biofilms. J Med Microbiol 1991; 48: 671-79.

[23] Costerton JW, Stewart PS, Greenberg EP. Bacterial biofilms: a common cause of persistent infections. Science1999; 284:1318-22.

[24] Mahenthiralingam E, Campbell ME, Speert DP. Non motility and phagocytic resistance of Pseudomonas aeruginosa isolates from chronically colonized patients with cystic fibrosis. Infect Immun 1994; 62: 596-605.

[25] Parsek MR, Singh PK. Bacterial biofilm: An emerging link to disease pathogenesis. Ann Rev Microbiol. 2003; 57: 677-701.

[26] Nickel JC, Olson M, McLean RJ, Grant SK, Costerton JW. An ecological study of infected urinary stone genesis in animal model. Br J Urol. 1987; 59: 21-30.

[27] Durack DT. Experimental bacterial endocarditis. IV. Structure and evolution of very early lesion. J Pathol. 1975; 115: 81-9.

[28] Koch C, Hoiby N. Pathogenesis of cystic fibrosis. Lancet 1993; 341: 1065-9.

[29] Govan JR, Deretic V. Microbial pathogenesis in cystic fibrosis: mucoid Pseudomonas aeruginosa and Burkolderia Cepacia. Microbiol Rev. 1996; 60 (3): 539-74.

[30] Marsh D. Microbiological ecology of dental plaque and its significance in health and disease. Adv Dent Res 1994;8: 263-271.

[31] Lamont RJ, Jenkinson HF. Life below gun line: pathogenic mechanism of Porphyromonas gingivalis. Microbiol Mol Biol Rev. 1998; 62: 1244-63.

[32] Usha HL, Kaiwar A, Mehta D. Biofilm in endodontics: New understanding to an old Problem. Int. journal of Contemporary Dentistry. 2010; 1(3): 44-51.

[33] Marrie TJ, Costerton JW. Mode of growth of bacterial pathogens in chronic polymicrobial human osteomyelitis. J Clin Microbiol. 1985; 22: 924-33.

[34] Nickel JC, Costerton JW. Bacterial localization in antibiotic-refractory chronic bacterial prostatis. Prostate 1993; 23: 107-114.

[35] Dart JKG. Contact lens and prosthesis infections. In Tasman W and Jager EA editors. Duane's foundation of Clinical ophthalmology. Lippincott-Raven, Pa: Philadelphia: 1996; p: 1-30.

[36] McLaughlin-Borlace L, Stapleton F, Matheson M, Dart JKG. Bacterial biofilm on contact lenses and lens storage cases in wearers with microbial keratitis. J Appl Microbiol. 1998;84: 827-38.

[37] Hancock EW. Artificial valve disease. In: Schtant RC, Alexander RW, Rourke RAO Roberts R and Sonnenblick EH, editors. The heart artiers and veins, 8th ed, vol. 2. New York: McGraw-Hill; NY. 1994. p:1539-45.

[38] Douglas JK, Cobbs CG. Prosthetic valve endocarditis In: Kaye D, editor. Infective endocarditis, 2nd ed. New York: Raven Press Ltd; N.Y. 1992. p: 375-396.

[39] Cramton SE, Gerke C, Schll NF, Nicholas WW, Gotz F. The intercellular adhesion (ica locus) is present in Staphylococcus aureus and is required for biofilm formation. Infect Immun. 1999; 67:5427-33.

[40] Heilmann C, Schweitzer O, Gerke C, Vanittanakom N, Mack D, Gotz F. Molecular basis of intercellular adhesions in the biofilm forming Staphylococcus epidermidis. Mol Microbiol. 1996; 20: 1083-91.

[41] National Nosocomial Infections Surveillance (NNIS) System Report. Data summary from January 1992 through June2004. Am Jinfect Control 2004; 32; 470-485.

[42] Warren JW. The catheter and urinary tract infection. Med Clin North Am1991; 75:481 - 493.

[43] Darouiche R, Device associated infections : A macroproblem that starts with microadherence. Clin. Infect Dis. 2001; 33: 1567-1572.

[44] Traunter BW and Darouiche RO. Catheter –associated infections: Pathogenesis affects Prevention. Arch Intern Med, 2004; 164: 842-850 .

[45] Lachman P and Yuen S. Using care bundles to prevent infection in neonatal and paediatric .ICUs. Curr. Opin infect Dis,2009; 22: 224-228.

[46] Fiel S. Guidelines and critical pathways for severe hospital- acquired pneumonia, Chest. 2011;119:412-418.

[47] Levis K. riddle of biofilm resistance. Antimicrob Agents Chemother 2001;45(4) : 999-1007.

[48] Brooun a, Liu S, Lewis K. A dose- response study of antibiotic resistance in Pseudomonas aeruginosa biofilms. Antimicrob Agents Chemother. 2000; 44; 640-646.

[49] Molin S, Tolker-Nielson T. Gene transfer occurs with enhanced efficiency in biofilms and induces enhanced stabilization of the biofilm structure. Curr Opin Biotechnol. 2003;14(3): 255-256.

[50] Shirtliff ME, Peters BM, Jabra-Rizk MA. Cross-kingdom intractions: Candida alicans and bacteria. FEMS Microbiol Lett. 2009; June:1-8.

[51] Peters BM, Jabra-Rizk MA, Scheper MA et al. Microbial interactions and differential protein expression in Staphylococcus aureus and Candida albicans dual-species biofilms. FEMS Imm Med Microbiol 2010; 59: 493-503.

[52] Harriott MM, Noverr MC. Candida albicans and Staphylococcus aureus form polymicrobial biofilms: effects on antimicrobial resistance. Antimicrob Agents Chemother. 2009; 53(9): 3914-3922.

[53] Hogan DA, Kolter R. Pseudomonas-Candida interactions: an ecological role for virulence factors. Science. 2002; 296(5576): 2229-2232.

[54] Costerton JW, Stewart PS, Greenberg EP. Bacterial biofilms: a common cause of persistentinfections. Science1999; 284:1318-1322.

[55] Washington CW Jr, Stephen DA, William MJ, Elmer WK, Gray WP, Paul CS, Gail LW. In Koneman's Colour Atlas and Textbook Of Diagnostic Microbiology, 6th ed, Lippincott Williams &Wilkins, Philadelphia PA, USA, 2006.

[56] Merritt JN, Kadouri DE, Toole G0. Grouping and analysing static biofilms. Ch Basic Protocol I,In current protocols in Microbiology, 2005; unit 1B. 1.1-1B.1.7

[57] Stepanovi s, Vukovi D, Daki I, Savib, Svabi-Vlahovi (M). A modified micotiter-plate test for quantitation of staphylococcal biofilm formation. JMicrobiol.Methods. 2000; 40:175- 179.

[58] Bose S, Khodke M, Basak S, Mallick S K. Detection of biofilm producing Staphylococci: Need of the hour. J. Clin and Diagnostic Res [serial online] 2009 December [cited: 2009 December 7]; 3:1915-1920. Available from http://www.jcdr.net/back asp?issn=0973-709x&year=2009&month= December &volume=3&issue=6&page=1915-1920 &id=469.

[59] Lee HW, Koh YM, Kim J et al Capacity of multidrug resistant clinical isolates of Acinetobacter baumanii to form biofilm and adhere to epithelial cell surfaces Clin. Microbiol Infect. 2008;14:49-54.

[60] norouzi F, Mansouri S, Moradi M, Razavi M Comparison of cell surface hydrophobicity and biofilm formation among ESBL and non ESBL producing Pseudomonas aeruginosa from clinical isolates. African Journal of Microbiology Research 2010;4(11):1143-1147.

[61] KhanF, Shukla I, Rizvi M, Mansoor T, Sharma SC Detection of biofilm formation in Staphylococcus aureus. Does it have a role in treatment of MRSA infections? Trends in Medical Research 2011;6:116-123.

[62] Spencer RC. Novel methods for prevention of infection of intravascular devices. J Hosp Infect. 1999; 43suppl: S127- 35.

[63] Johansen C, Falholt P, Gram L. Engymatic removal and disinfection of bacterial biofilm. Appl Enviorn Mirobial. 1997; 63: 3724-8.

[64] Maki DG, Ringer M, Alvarado CJ Prospective randomized trial of povidone iodine, alcohol and chlorhexidine for prevention of infection associated with central venous and arterial catheters. Lancet 1991;338:339-343.

[65] Curtin J, Cormican M, Fleming G, Keeiehan J, Colleran E Linezolid compared with eperezolid, vancomycin and gentamicin in an in vitro model of antimicrobial lock

therapy for Staphylococcus epidermidis central venous catheter related biofilm infections. Antimicrobial. Agents Chemother. 2003;47:3145-3148.

[66] Curtin JJ and Donlan RM Using bacteriophages to reduce formation of catheter associated biofilms by Staphylococcus epidermidis. Antimicrobial. Agents Chemother. 2006;50(4):1268-1275.

[67] Vejborg RM and Klemm P Blocking of bacterial biofilm formation by a fish protein coating Appl.Environ.Microbiol. 2008.

[68] Blenkinsopp SA, Khoury AE, Costerion JW Electrical enhancement of biocide efficacy against Pseudomonas aeruginosa biofilms. Appl. Envioron.Microbiol. 1992;58:3770-3773.

[69] Huang CT, James G, Pitt WG, Stewart PS Effects of ultrasonic treatment on the efficacy of gentamicin against established Pseudomonas aeruginosa biofilms. Colloids Surfaces B Bioineterfaces 1996;6:235-242.

[70] Hartman G, Wise R. Quonum sensing. Potential means of treating Gram negative infection? Lancet 1998; 351: 848-9.

Chapter 4

Ocular Infections Caused by *Corynebacterium* Species

Hiroshi Eguchi

Additional information is available at the end of the chapter

http://dx.doi.org/10.5772/56214

1. Introduction

1.1. The history of *Corynebacterium* species

The most well-known *Corynebacterium* species, *Corynebacterium diphtheliae,* causes diphtheria. However, in 1970, the clinical value of identification of *Corynebacterium* diphtheriae became less medically significant owing to the development of diphtheria toxoids and a decrease in the prevalence of diphtheritic infection in developed countries. Other *Corynebacterium* species have been considered contaminants when found in clinical samples because they are organisms normally found in the skin, mucous membranes, and other human tissues. Given that *Corynebacterium* species are one of the most commonly isolated bacteria from the ocular surfaces [1, 2], they are also considered non-pathogenic in the ophthalmic field.

Currently, in a clinical setting, many bacteriological laboratory technicians in hospitals report *Corynebacterium* species as "Gram-positive rods". Sometimes, the presence of *Corynebacterium* species is not reported because it is considered to be contaminants. As a result, it is not possible for ophthalmologists to determine whether *Corynebacterium* species are present in clinical samples by using laboratory tests. This makes the *Corynebacterium* species to be nonpathogenic for ophthalmologists leading to therapeutic failure.

2. Bacteriological characteristics of *Corynebacterium* species

Morphology: The size of *Corynebacterium* species varies from 0.3–0.8 × 1–8 μm. They exsist in a variety of shapes, even in pure cultures. In the clinical samples, they mostly appear as rod-shaped bacteria in palisade-, ring-, or 'I, N, T, V, W, or Y' letter-shaped arrangments.

Lipophilicity: Few *Corynebacterium* species generally have high lipophilicity. In vitro, they can be easily become unculturable if the final concentration of Tween 80 (polysorbate 80) in the medium is slightly different from the optimal concentration. Presumably, this is the reason why particular *Corynebacterium* species prefer the ocular surfaces as these are area where fatty acids are always present because they are secreted from the meibomian gland. This requirement may also explain why *Corynebacterium*-induced endophthalmitis is very rare.

3. *Corynebacterium* species as a pathogen: Case presentations

Case 1: In 2003, the author encountered the case of an elderly patient who had clear infectious conjunctivitis in his right eye. He had experienced mild conjunctival hyperaemia and mucopurulent discharge after cataract surgery performed 2 years before consultation (Fig. 1). He had continued to use a quinolone ophthalmic solution postoperatively, but had not undergone any ophthalmic examination. He had eye discomfort for more than 3 months. Gram staining smear of the discharge showed that many polymorphonuclear leukocytes phagocytizing Gram-positive rods (Fig. 2). Culture of the discharge sample detected quinolone resistant *Corynebacterium* species, and the strain was susceptible to cephem antibiotics. Switching the quinolone ophthalmic solution to a cephem antibiotic resolved of the patient's symptoms. The author determined this to be a clear case of conjunctivitis due to *Corynebacterium* species. Thereafter, the author encountered a large number of cases of *Corynebacterium* conjunctivitis in geriatric patient as well as several cases of *Corynebacterium* keratitis in patients who underwent keratoplasty. Thus, in 2012, *Corynebacterium* species still appear to be pathogens of the ocular surface.

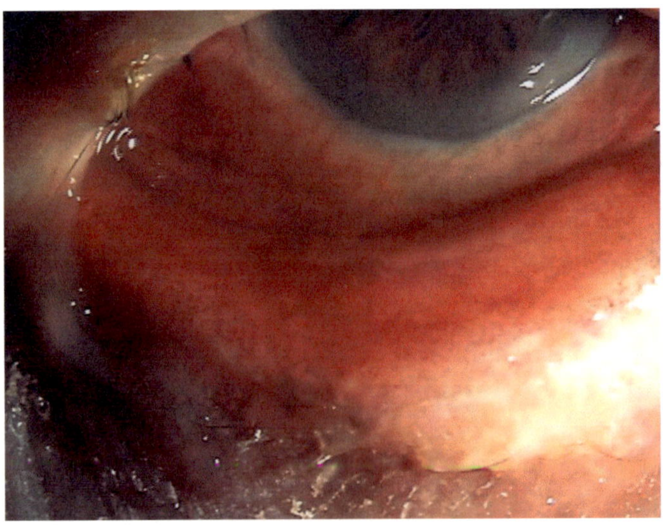

Figure 1. Infectious conjunctivitis occurred in case 1. A mild infectious conjunctivitis was found.

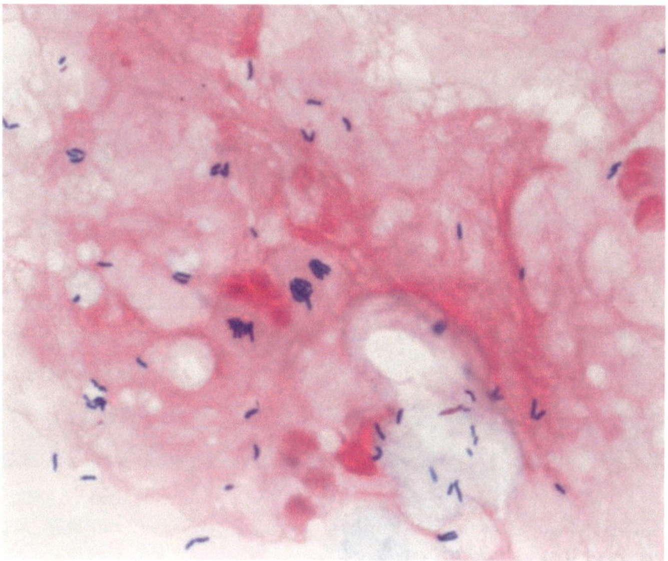

Figure 2. Gram stain of the discharge sample from case 1, original magnification ×1000 Gram-positive rods shaped bacteria in palisade- and 'I, or V' letter-shaped formations were found within polymorphonuclear neutrophil leukocytes.

Case 2: Figures 3 A & B show an ocular surface of a diabetic young man. He had intractable filamentous keratitis after 2 vitrectomies. When he was referred to the author's clinic, a moxifloxacin ophthalmic solution has been prescribed for more than 6 months (from the perioperative stage of the first vitrectomy). After the diagnosis of infectious blepharoconjunctivitis with mucopurulent yellowish discharge, it was determined that the blepharoconjunctivitis may have caused swelling of the eyelid, and the swollen eyelid partially induced intractable filamentous keratitis. Analysis of a smear of the discharge showed a large number of polymorphonuclear leukocytes and Gram-positive rod-shaped bacteria in palisade- and 'I, V, or W' letter-shaped arrangements (Fig. 4). *Corynebacterium* species were identified in the culture of the discharge by using a simple, commercially available identification kit (BBL Crystal, BD, Japan, Tokyo). The author also isolated *Corynebacterium* species on a sheep blood agar plate from the discharge and identified the causative agent as *Corynebacterium macginleyi* on the basis of its biochemical characters tested by API-Coryne (bioMérieux SA, Lyon, France). The minimum inhibitory concentration (MIC) of moxifloxacin and ceftriaxone for the strain (tested by E-test®, bioMérieux SA, Lyon, France) was >256μg/mL and 2 μg/mL, respectively. Switching moxifloxacin to topical cephmenoxim led to rapid improvement of blepharoconjunctivitis and filamentous keratitis (Fig. 5).

It is currently no exaggeration to say that *Corynebacterium* species are among the major pathogens responsible for chronic conjunctivitis, especially in geriatric patients. These pathogens can also cause infectious keratitis in patients who are immune-compromised [3-5]. All such conditions may be triggered, when the bacterial flora of the ocular surface are disturbed, by opportunistic infections. Endophthalmitis caused by *Corynebacterium* species is

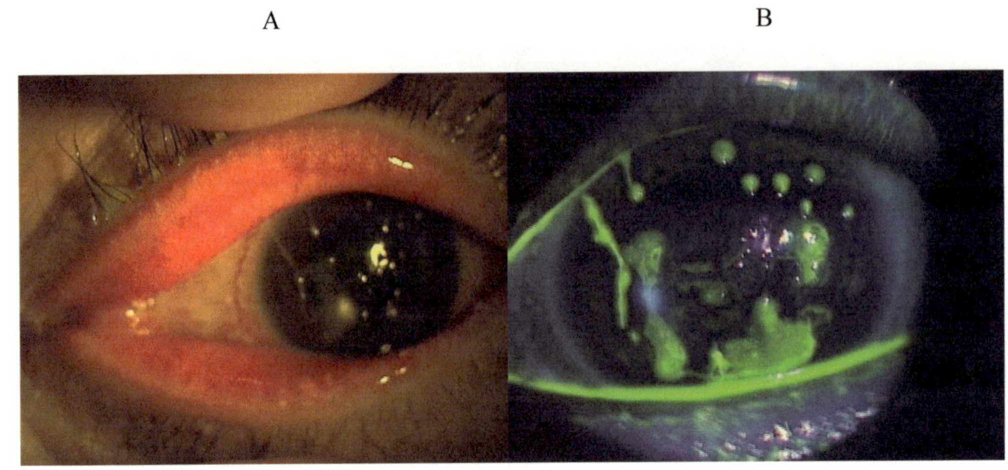

Figure 3. Anterior segments of case 2. Moderate blepharoconjunctivitis, yellowish mucopurulent discharge, and corneal erosion with filamentous keratitis were found.

very rare. Although *C. macginleyi* is the common *Corynebacterium* species to be isolated from the ocular surface [6, 7], it remains unclear whether *C. macginleyi* is the major species responsible for ocular infections because cases caused by other species have been documented as well [5].

4. Diagnostic techniques

According to Koch's postulates, when establishing the specificity of a pathogenic microorganism, the first criterion is the organism must be present in all cases of the disease. Although quantitative analysis of a specific bacterium in samples by using real-time polymerase chain reaction may be useful, this technique is not readily available to practitioners. It is difficult to validate the other criteria of Koch's postulate, always in clinical setting. Thus, most clinical ophthalmologists depend only on first criterion when identifying a pathogen.

The first step when diagnosing and treating *Corynebacterium* infections should be to subject the clinical samples, such as mucopurulent discharge or corneal scrapings, to Gram staining, examine them microscopically, and observe whether Gram-positive rods suggestive of *Corynebacterium* species appear ingested by polymorphonuclear leukocytes (Fig. 2, 4). Finally, the culture results must be accounted.

Although the culture results from discharge and corneal scrapings have clinical significance, we should also recognize the risk of overestimation. As a proof of this, the author has received culture results identifying *Staphylococcus epidermidis* as a pathogen even though plenty of Gram-positive rods are normally found on microscopy in some patients. In some cases,

http://dx.doi.org/10.5772/56214

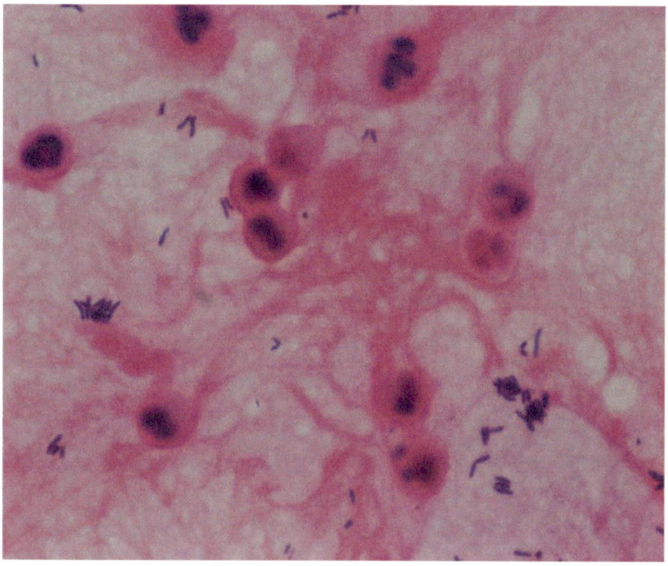

Figure 4. Gram stain of the discharge sample from case 2, original magnification ×1000 A large number of Gram-positive rods are phagocytised by polymorphonuclear neutrophil leukocytes.

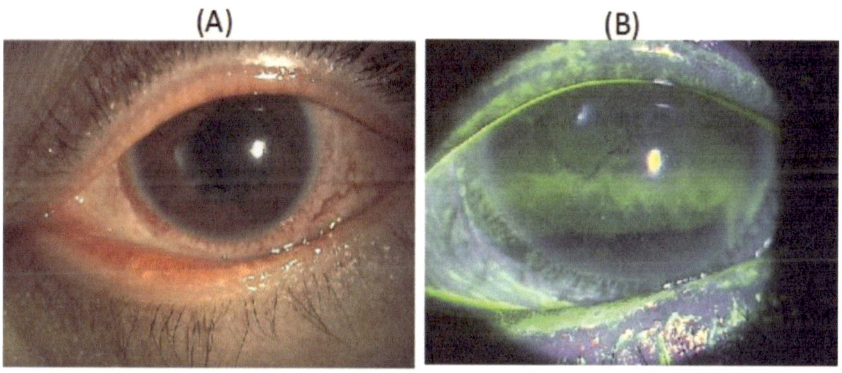

Figure 5. Post-medication. The blepharoconjunctivitis and filamentous keratitis are disappeared.

a 'culture negative' result is reported. Figure 6 shows the anterior segments of a bedridden elderly female patient (A) and a panorama Gram stain image of her eye discharge (B). She had a conjunctival hyperaemia with a large amount of yellowish white mucopurulent discharge that lasted for 1 week. The smear prepared from discharge was stained by Gram staining, which showed a large amount of Gram-postitive rods suggestive of *Corynebacterium* species. Although she clearly had infectious conjunctivitis and no medication had been administered, the culture result from her discharge was reported as negative. Hence, the smear and microscopic examination of clinical samples contribute significantly to the diagnosis of ocular infections caused by *Corynebacterium* species.

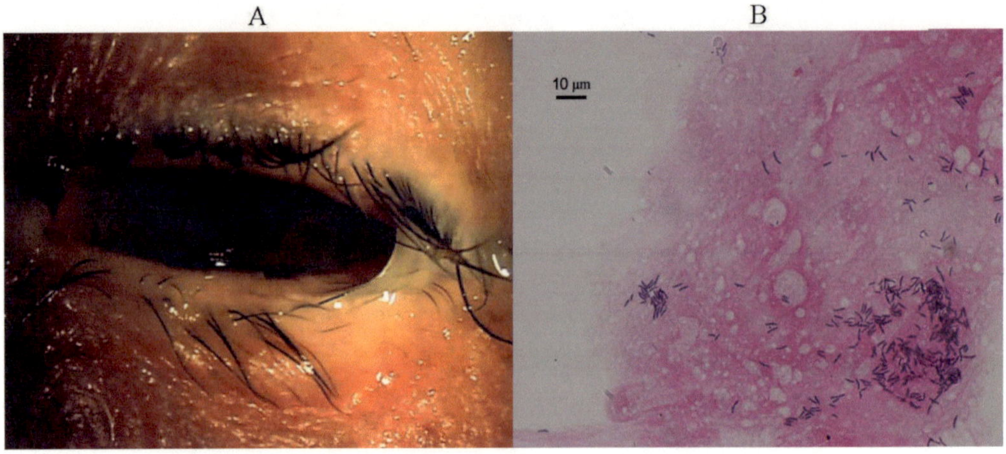

Figure 6. Severe infectious conjunctivitis and a Gram-stained panoramic image of the discharge sample. A: A large quantity of yellowish-white mucopurulent discharge and conjunctival hyperaemia were found. B: A large amount of Gram-positive rods and a few polymorphonuclear leukocytes were found.

Antimicrobial	Max MIC	Min MIC	% Susceptible*
Nolfloxacin	256	0.25	25
Ciprofloxacin	32	0.032	25
Levofloxacin	32	0.064	25
Gatifloxacin	32	0.016	40
Moxifloxacin	32	0.016	40
Erythromycin	256	0.016	45
Chloramphenicol	256	2	55
Gentamicin	16	0.064	95
Tobramycin	32	0.064	90
Doxycycline	4	0.064	100
Imipenem	0.08	0.016	100
Ceftriaxson	0.5	0.125	100
Vancomycin	0.5	1	100
Teicoplanin	0.125	1	100

*: The susceptibility test follow the instruction of E-test.

Table 1. MICs of several antimicrobials to 20 bacterial strains. (μg/mL)

http://dx.doi.org/10.5772/56214

5. Observation and result

The author found that *Corynebacterium* species isolated from the ocular surfaces of elderly patients in Japan are very sensitive to cephem antibiotics (Table 1, unpublished data). Although they are also sensitive to aminoglycosides, most of the strains are highly resistant to quinolone [7].

6. Conclusion

When faced with the case of an elderly patient with chronic conjunctivitis, the first step should be to collect the discharge and to prepare a Gram stained smear and observation under microscope. Assessment should also determine whether the lacrimal duct is obstructed or not. Documenting a patient's history of antimicrobial use will also contribute to the diagnosis. If the patient has a history of using an antimicrobial ophthalmic solution, and also has Gram-positive rods in palisade, ring or 'N, T, V, W, or Y' letter-shaped arrangement present in their discharge and if these Gram positive rods appear to be ingested by polymorphonuclear leukocytes, then a cephem-based ophthalmic solution should be prescribed first. It is possible that an organism other than a *Corynebacterium* species is the causative pathogen if the cephem antibiotics do not resolve the infection. For *Corynebacterium*-induced keratitis, a systemic carbapenem and glycopeptide may be useful in additions to frequent applications of cephem, aminoglycoside, and glycopeptide eye drops.

Author details

Hiroshi Eguchi*

Address all correspondence to: hiroegu@clin.med.tokushima-u.ac.jp

Department of Ophthalmology, Institute of Health Biosciences, The University of Tokushima Graduate School, Tokushima-shi, Japan

References

[1] Inoue Y, Usui M, Ohashi Y, et al. Preoperative disinfection of the conjunctival sac with antibiotics and iodine compound: a prospective randomized multicenter study. Jpn J Ophthalmol. 2008; 52: 151-161

[2] Hara J, Yasuda F, Higashitsutsumi M.Ophthalmologica1997; 211(suppl 1): 62-67

[3] Suzuki T, Ihara H, Uno T, et al. Suture-related keratitis caused by Corynebacterium-macginleyi. J Clin Microbiol. 2007; 45:3833-3836

[4] Fukumoto A, Sotozono C, Hieda O, et al. Infectious keratitis caused by fluoroquinolone-resistant Corynebacterium. Jpn J Ophthalmol. 2011;55:579-580

[5] Inada K, Maeda I, Miyazaki D, et al. A case of infectious keratitis caused by Corynebacterium. Atrashii Gannka (in Japanese) 2009; 26:1105-1107

[6] Funke G, Pagano-Niedere M, Bernaucer W. Corynebacterium macginleyi has to date been isolated exclusively from conjunctival swabs. J Clin Microbiol. 1998; 36:3670-3673

[7] Eguchi H, Kuwahara T, Miyamoto T, et al. High-level fluoroquinolone resistance in ophthalmic clinical isolates belonging to the species Corynebacterium macginleyi. J Clin Microbiol. 2008; 46:527-532

Chapter 5

Acinetobacter

Lul Raka, Gjyle Mulliqi-Osmani, Lumturije Begolli,
Arsim Kurti, Greta Lila, Rrezarta Bajrami and
Arbëresha Jaka-Loxha

Additional information is available at the end of the chapter

http://dx.doi.org/10.5772/55618

1. Introduction

Infections caused by bacteria of genus Acinetobacter pose a significant health care challenge worldwide (Munoz-Price & Weinstein, 2008; Visca et al., 2011). Acinetobacter infections in the past were sporadically identified in hospitalized patients and hospital infection outbreaks in intensive care units. But, nowadays Acinetobacter has emerged as an important healthcare-associated and multidrug-resistant microorganism (Peleg at al., 2008).

Acinetobacter was first described in 1911 by Beijerinck as Micrococcus calco-aceticus. The name "Acinetobacter" originates from the Greek word "akinetos" meaning "unable to move", as these bacteria are not motile. A. baumannii, A. calcoaceticus, A. haemolyticus and A. lwoffii are the most important species in clinical practice.

Acinetobacter species are ubiquitous in nature and have been found in soil, water, animals and humans. Some strains of Acinetobacter can survive for weeks in environment, promoting transmission within the hospital settings (Doughari et al., 2011). Acinetobacter baumannii was recovered from the skin, throat, rectum and respiratory tract of humans. The species A. baumannii accounts for nearly 80% of reported Acinetobacter infections (CDC,2007). This feature along with antimicrobial resistance, colonization potential and contact transmission are main challenges for prevention and control activities (Maragakis et al., 2008). Some strains of Acinetobacter produce verotoxins and others have been identified to have an impact on removal of biological phosphorus from wastewater.

2. Taxonomy and main features

Genus Acinetobacter belongs to the family Moraxellaceae and order Pseudomonadales.

Based on molecular studies, 32 species of Acinetobacter have now been recognized; 22 of them have assigned valid names, whereas other species are described as a "genomic" group. The most important clinical species in medicine is Acinetobacter baumannii. This micro-organism has phenotypicall similarities with a group of species known as A.calcoaceticus-A.baumannii complex (Vaneechoutte et al., 2011). In healthcare settings, this group is implicated in major outbreaks and healthcare-associated infections.

The genus Acinetobacter consists of strictly aerobic Gram-negative coccobacilli rods, which are nonmotile, catalase-positive, indole-negative, oxidase-negative, non-fermentative. The bacilli are 0.9 to 1.6 μm in diameter and 1.5 to 2.5 μm in length, often in pairs or assembled into longer chains. Acinetobacter spp. are non-fastidious and can be grown on standard laboratory media.

Acinetobacter is relatively nonreactive in many biochemical tests used to differentiate among gram-negative bacilli. Most clinical microbiology laboratories identify members of the genus Acinetobacter at the level of the following three groups with corresponding metabolic attributes (Allen et al., 2006):

- Acinetobacter calcoaceticus-baumannii complex: glucose-oxidizing non-hemolytic (A.baumannii can be identified by OXA-51 serotyping)
- Acinetobacter lwoffii: non glucose-oxidizing, non-hemolytic
- Acinetobacter haemolyticus: hemolytic.

http://dx.doi.org/10.5772/55618

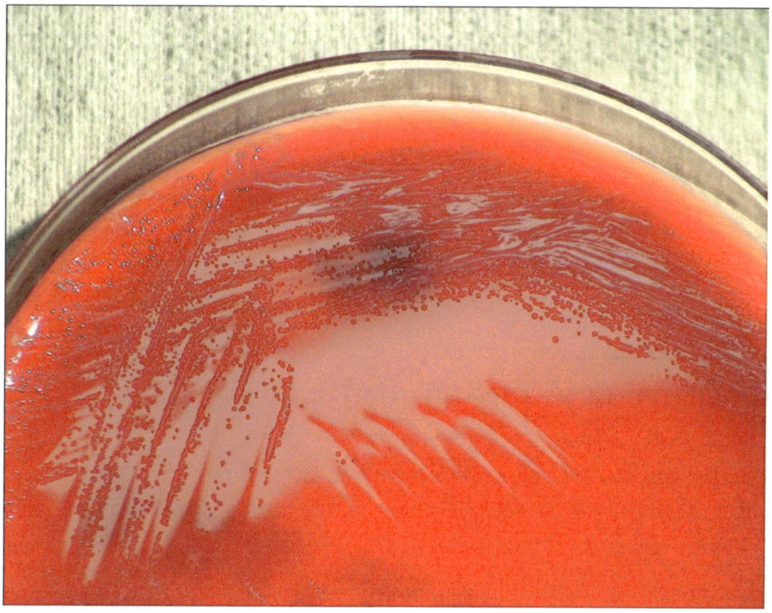

Figure 1. Colonies of Acinetobacter spp. on sheep's blood agar after 24 hours at 37°C. CDC/ Pete Seidel. Public Health Image Library

Acinetobacter species are widely distributed in nature and can be found in soil, sewage, water, consumables (including fruits and vegetables), and on healthy skin and other body sites. A. baumannii can be found also in some unusual reservoirs, such as food or arthropods. The majority of A. baumannii strains survive longer than Escherichia coli on dry surfaces, and some strains survive for more than 4 months.

About 25% of adults carry this organism on their skin, whereas about 7% carry it in their pharynx. Hospitalized patients may become easily colonized. Half of the patients with tracheostomy may be colonized with Acientobacter. Isolation of this microorganism from feces, urine, vaginal secretions is often considered as colonization or contamination. But, their presence from immunocompromised persons may have significant clinical impact (Mahon et al., 2010).

Clinical infections with Acinetobacter in healthcare settings are related to the use of invasive procedures (mechanical ventilation, vascular catheters) and patient's underlying conditions (Fournier & Richet, 2006). The most important risk factors for acquiring Acinetobacter infections are: prior antibiotic use (third-generation cephalosporins, fluoroquinolones or carbapenems), prolonged hospitalization, high APACHE II (Acute Physiology and Chronic Health Evaluation) score, recent surgical intervention, central vascular catheterization, tracheostomy, mechanical ventilation and enteral feeding.

Acinetobacter can contaminate many surfaces and medical equipment, such are: suctioning equipment, washbasins, bedrails, bedside tables, ventilators, sinks, pillows, mattresses, hygroscopic bandages, resuscitation equipment, and trolleys (Bernards et al., 2004). The hands of healthcare workers are in frequent contact with these objects in patient surroundings. Hands become an important vectors of transmission in case of non-compliance with hand hygiene recommendations (Pittet et al., 2006). The ability of Acinetobacter to participate in biofilm formation promotes durability in surfaces and may contribute to continuation of environmental presence during outbreaks (Fournier et al., 2006).

Acinetobacter species posses the following virulence factors which enable transmission within health care settings: cell surface hydrophobicity, enzymes, toxic slime polysaccharides, verotoxins, siderophores and outer membrane proteins.

3. Clinical importance — Infections and outbreaks

Acinetobacter spp. can cause infections in both hospital settings and in community. They are the second most commonly isolated non-fermenters in human specimens, after Pseudomonas aeruginosa. About 1-3% of health care-associated infections are caused by Acientobacter spp.

Acinetobacter poses little risk to healthy people. However, people who have weakened immune systems, chronic lung disease, or diabetes may be more susceptible to infections with Acinetobacter. Most infections caused by this multiresistant bacteria involve organ systems, which have a high fluid content (the respiratory tract, peritoneal fluid, and the urinary tract) and are associated with usage of indwelling devices. The distribution of the different types of hospital acquired infections is variable between hospitals and it depends on the hospital population and the type of performed procedures and interventions. Rates of mortality from Acinetobacter infections have a wide range from 5% in general wards to 54% in intensive care units (Kempf & Rolain, 2012).

One important feature of A. baumannii is its ability to cause outbreaks, which is in relation to antimicrobial resistance and resistance to desiccation (D'Agata et al., 2000; Villegas et Hartstein, 2003). Acinetobacter spp. cause a wide range of health care-associated infections such as: ventilator-associated pneumonia, bloodstream infections, urinary tract infections, surgical site infections, meningitis, cholangitis, peritonitis, skin and wound infections, ventriculitis, and infective endocarditis. Suppuration is common feature in infections caused by Acientobacter (abscesses of the brain, lung and the thyroid; secondary infections of wounds or surgical trauma, and purulent lesions of the eye).

Acinetobacter can also cause infections in the community (Falagas et al., 2007). The predominant community-acquired infections are: pneumonia, meningitis, cellulitis and bacteremia. High fatality rates in community were correlated to underlying conditions and risk factors, such as : alcoholism, diabetes and cancer.

Acinetobacter infections were also frequently reported during the natural disasters and wars (Iraq, Kuwait and Afghanistan wars). Pathogenic Acinetobacter infections were encountered in military personnel during the wars in Afghanistan and Iraq (O'Shea, 2012).Therefore it was named by media as Iraqibacter.

Recent disasters suggested that Acinetobacter infections should be taken in consideration in differential diagnosis of soft-tissue infections (Asia tsunami on 2004).

Many Acinetobacter infections have a seasonal variation with 50% infection rates higher from July to October than at other times of the year. This variation was explained by warmer, more humid ambient air, which favors growth of Acinetobacter and potentially preventable environmental contaminants, such as condensate from air-conditioners.

4. Antimicrobial resistance

The main challenge with A. baumannii is it's ability to acquire antimicrobial-resistance genes extremely rapidly, leading to multidrug resistance. Widespread use of antimicrobials within hospitals resulted to the emergence and increase of antimicrobial resistance among Acinetobacter strains, in particular, the wide use of extended-spectrum cephalosporins and quinolones (Imperi et al, 2011).

Acinetobacter spp. are intrinsically less susceptible to antimicrobial agents than other representatives from the family Enterobacteriaceae. Various mechanisms played a role in the acquisition of a multiresistance phenotype amongst Gram-negative bacteria, including Acinetobacter strains such as: loss of porins, production of β-lactamases, increased expression of efflux pumps, presence of antibiotic-modifying enzymes, target site mutations, ribosomal mutations or modifications, metabolic bypass mechanisms and a mutation in the lipopolysaccharide (Poirel et al, 2011). The role of plasmids in the acquisition of antimicrobial resistance in A. baumannii is mostly related to their integron structures.

Acinetobacter spp have ability to acquire antimicrobial-resistance genes rapidly, leading to multidrug resistance. As a result, the clinical management of these infections has become a public health challenge in many countries. Nowadays, the most serious problem in the treatment of Acinetobacter infection is acquired multidrug-resistance, leaving only few antimicrobial agents as treatment options. This resistance is attributed to the presence of multiple resistant determinant among bacteria, which confers resistance to many groups of antimicrobial agents (Livermore, 2012). One of the main concerns about antimicrobial resistance in A.baumannii has been the resistance to the last line of antimicrobials through acquisition of carbapenem resistance - mainly through the acquisition of B and D class carbapenemases(Bou et al., 2012).

5. Detection and typing systems

Infection or colonization with Acinetobacter is usually diagnosed by the culture of clinical samples and samples from environment. The most frequent clinical samples include blood, cerebrospinal fluid, endotracheal aspirate, wounds, sputum, urine, catheter tips, stool or sterile body fluid, skin, cordon of newborns, nasal swabs, hand swabs of hospital workers. The most common environmental samples include swabs on surfaces of machines, wash-hand basins, floors, tables, UV lamps, etc.

Microbiologic cultures can be processed by standard methods on routine media. For routine clinical and laboratory investigations, traditional culture media are used: agar, brain heart infusion agar, tryptic soy agar, Eosin-methylene blue, MacConkey agar, Violet red bile agar, Luria Bertani agar and Holton medium. For environmental screening the most commonly used media are broth media such as MacConkey's broth, trypton soy, Brain Heart Infusion and Luria broth. Antimicrobial susceptibility can be determined by various means, with the agar-dilution method being the gold-standard (CLSI, 2011).

Biochemical typing methods include the use of colorimetric based GN card ID 32 GN, API 20NE, RapID NF Plus and Vitek 2 systems.

For detection of Acinetobacter strains a new molecular identification and typing methods have been developed, leading to successful identification and outbreak management (Ecker et al., 2006). The most important of them are : polymerase chain reaction (PCR), PFGE, RAPD-PCR DNA fingerprinting, fluorescent in situ hybridization (FISH), 16S rRNA gene restriction analysis (ARDRA) (amplified rDNA restriction analysis) and 16S rRNA gene PCR-DGGE (Denaturing Gradient Gel Electrophoresis) fingerprinting (Versalovic et al., 2011). A recent diagnostic method which was reported to have high specificity and can discriminate between Acinetobacter species is the microsphere-based array technique that combines an allele specific primer extension assay and microsphere hybridization. The use of DNA-DNA hybridization and sequence analysis is considered the gold standard, but the method is time consuming and impractical in most clinical laboratories.

Other methods that have been introduced in the epidemiological investigation of outbreaks caused by Acinetobacter spp. include biotyping, phage typing, cell envelope protein typing, plasmid typing, ribotyping, restriction fragment length polymorphisms and arbitrarily primed PCR (AP-PCR).

6. Treatment, prevention and control

Treatment of Acinetobacter infections should be individualized according to results of susceptibility testings. For effective treatment of Acinetobacter infections the combination therapy is usually required. Infections caused by antibiotic-susceptible Acinetobacter isolates have usually been treated with broad-spectrum cephalosporins, combinations of β-lactam:β-lactamase inhibitor or carbapenems, used alone or in combination with an aminoglycoside (Evans et al., 2012). The duration of treatment is similar to that for infections caused by other gram-negative bacilli.

Antibiotic choices may be limited in cases of infections caused by multidrug-resistant isolates. The emergence of multidrug-resistant Acinetobacter strains has brought the old antibiotic polymyxins back into clinical use. These antibiotics disrupt bacterial cytoplasmic membranes, causing leakage of cytoplasmic contents. Clinicians stoped using this antibiotic in 1970s due to several side effects in kidneys and neurons.

http://dx.doi.org/10.5772/55618

Another treatment option remain tigecycline, a new glycylcycline antibiotic. However, development of resistance to these last option antibiotics has been reported recently (Gimarellou & Poulakou, 2012).

Prevention and control of infections caused by Acinetobacter requires a coordinated effort involving all stakeholders including healthcare facilities and providers, public health, and industry (Siegel et al., 2007). CDC and APIC has recommend the cornerstones for prevention and control of multidrug resistant organisms, including Acinetobacter infections (CDC,2012; APIC,2010). Key measures to control spread of multi-drug resistant organisms are:

- Administrative Measures/Adherence Monitoring
- Education
- Judicious Antimicrobial Use
- Surveillance
- Infection Control Precautions to Prevent Transmission
- Environmental Measures Decolonization

Infection control measures should start with strict isolation and cohorting of infected or colonized patients accompanied by administrative measures, education, prudent antimicrobial use, surveillance, standard precautions to prevent transmission and environmental measures.

Control of hospital outbreaks caused by Acinetobacter species is an important challenge for all health care settings. If a source and/or reservoir are identified, than the outbreak is successfully controlled by the eradication of that source/reservoir. In other circumstances, various measures may be used, including unit closure, cohorting of patients and staff, strict hand hygiene, contact or strict isolation, environmental disinfection and discharge of colonized patients.

A review of 51 hospital outbreaks showed that 25 had a common source: 13 outbreaks with predominantly respiratory tract infections and 12 with predominantly bloodstream or other infections were controlled by removal or disinfection and sterilization of contaminated ventilator (or related) equipment or contaminated moist fomites (Villegas & Hartstein, 2003).

When neither common sources nor environmental reservoirs are identified, control has depended on active surveillance and contact isolation for colonized and infected patients, improvements in the hand hygiene of health care workers and aseptic care of vascular catheters and endotracheal tubes.

7. Conclusions

In conclusion, Acinetobacter strains are important pathogens due to the diversity of their reservoirs, capacity to accumulate mechanisms of antimicrobial resistance and outbreak potential. Acinetobacter infections prolong the length of hospital stay, increase mortality and have economic impact. The greatest challenge remain prevention, control and treatment of infections caused by multidrug-resistant strains of Acinetobacter.

Although our understanding of Acinetobacter made an significant step forward, there are still many unanswered questions for health care workers. Future directions should be directed toward research development of new antibiotics, well-controlled clinical trials of antimicrobial regimens and combinations, and prevention of health care-associated transmission of multi-drug-resistant Acinetobacter infections.

Author details

Lul Raka, Gjyle Mulliqi-Osmani, Lumturije Begolli, Arsim Kurti, Greta Lila, Rrezarta Bajrami and Arbëresha Jaka-Loxha

*Address all correspondence to: lul.raka@uni-pr.edu lulraka@hotmail.com

Faculty of Medicine, University of Prishtina & National Institute of Public Health of Kosova, Prishtina, Kosova

References

[1] Allen, S, Procop, G, & Schreckenberger, P. Guidelines for the collection, transport, processing, analysis, and reporting of cultures from specific specimen sources. In: Winn WC, Koneman EE, eds. Koneman's Color Atlas and Textbook of Diagnostic Microbiology. 4th ed. Philadelphia: Lippincott Williams & Wilkins; (2006)., 68-105.

[2] Bernards, A. T. Harinck HIJ, Dijkshoorn L, van der Reijden TJK, van den Broek PJ. Persistent Acinetobacter baumannii? Look inside your medical equipment. Infect Control Hosp Epidemiol. (2004)., 25, 1002-1004.

[3] Bou, G, Otero, F. M, Santiso, R, Tamayo, M, Fernández, M. D, Tomás, M, Gosálvez, J, & Fernández, J. L. Fast Assessment of Resistance to Carbapenem and Ciprofloxacin of Clinical Strains of Acinetobacter baumannii. J Clin Microbiol. (2012)., 50, 3609-13.

[4] Clinical and Laboratory Standards Institute [Internet]Performance Standards for Antimicrobial Susceptibility Testing; Twenty-First Informational Supplement. CLSI document MS21. (2011). updated 2011 Jul 8; cited 2012 Sep 23]. Available from: http://www.clsi.org/source/orders/free/m100-s19.pdf, 100.

[5] Cohen, A, et al. Recommendations for metrics for multidrug-resistant organisms in healthcare settings: SHEA/HICPAC Position Paper. Infect Control Hosp Epidemiol. (2008)., 29, 1099-1106.

[6] D'Agata EMC, Thayer V, Schaffner W. An Outbreak of Acinetobacter baumannii: The Importance of Cross-Transmission. Infect Control Hosp Epidemiol. 2000;21:588-591.

[7] Davis, K. A, Moran, K. A, Mcallister, C. K, & Gray, P. G. Multidrug-resistant Acinetobacter extremity infections in soldiers. Emerg Infect Dis. (2005). , 11, 1218-1224.

[8] Doughari, H, Ndakiedemi, P, Human, I, & Benade, S. The Ecology, Biology and Pathogenesis of Acinetobacter spp.: An Overview. Microbes Environ. (2011). , 26(2), 101-112.

[9] Ecker, J. A, Massire, C, Hall, T. A, et al. Identification of Acinetobacter species and genotyping of Acinetobacter baumannii by multilocus PCR and mass spectrometry. J Clin Microbiol. (2006). , 44(8), 2921-2932.

[10] Evans, B. A, Hamouda, A, & Amyes, S. G. The Rise of Carbapenem-Resistant Acinetobacter baumannii. Curr Pharm Des. (2012).

[11] Falagas, M. E, Karveli, E. A, Kelesidis, I, & Kelesidis, T. Community-acquired Acinetobacter infections. Eur J Clin Microbiol Infect Dis. (2007). , 26(12), 857-868.

[12] Fournier, P, Vallenet, D, & Barbe, V. et. al. Comparative Genomics of Multidrug Resistance in Acinetobacter baumannii. PLoS Genet. (2006). , 2, 62-72.

[13] Fournier, P. E, & Richet, H. The epidemiology and control of Acinetobacter baumannii in health care facilities. Clin Infect Dis. (2006). , 42(5), 692-699.

[14] Giamarellou, H, & Poulakou, G. Pharmacokinetic and pharmacodynamic evaluation of tigecycline. Expert Opin Drug Metab Toxicol. (2011). , 7(11), 1459-70.

[15] Guide to the Elimination of Multidrug-resistant Acinetobacter baumannii Transmission in Healthcare SettingsAPIC Guide (2010).

[16] Imperi, F, Antunes, L. C, Blom, J, Villa, L, Iacono, M, Visca, P, & Carattoli, A. The genomics of Acinetobacter baumannii: insights into genome plasticity, antimicrobial resistance and pathogenicity. IUBMB Life. (2011). Dec;, 63(12), 1068-74.

[17] Kempf, M, & Rolain, J. M. Emergence of resistance to carbapenems in Acinetobacter baumannii in Europe: clinical impact and therapeutic options. Int J Antimicrob Agents. (2012). , 39(2), 105-14.

[18] Livermore, D. M. Fourteen years in resistance. Int J Antimicrob Agents. (2012). , 39(4), 283-94.

[19] Maragakis, L. L, & Perl, T. M. Acinetobacter baumannii: epidemiology, antimicrobial resistance, and treatment options. Clin Infect Dis. (2008). Apr 15;, 46(8), 1254-1263.

[20] Shea, O. MK. Acinetobacter in modern warfare. Int J Antimicrob Agents. (2012). May;, 39(5), 363-75.

[21] Peleg, A. Y, Seifert, H, & Paterson, D. L. Acinetobacter baumannii: emergence of a successful pathogen. Clin Microbiol Rev. (2008). Jul;, 21(3), 538-582.

[22] Pittet, D, Allegranzi, B, Sax, H, et al. Evidence-based model for hand transmission during patient care and the role of improved practices. Lancet Infect Dis. (2006). , 6, 641-652.

[23] Poirel, L, Bonnin, R. A, & Nordmann, P. Genetic basis of antibiotic resistance in pathogenic Acinetobacter species. IUBMB Life. (2011). Dec;, 63(12), 1061-7.

[24] Siegel, J. D, Rhinehart, E, Jackson, M, & Chiarello, L. Healthcare Infection Control Practices Advisory Committee. 2007. Guideline for isolation precautions: preventing transmission of infectious agents in health care settings. Am J Infect Control. (2007). Dec;35(10 Suppl 2):S, 65-164.

[25] Silvia Munoz-Price LWeinstein RA. Acinetobacter Infection. N Engl J Med (2008). , 358, 1271-81.

[26] Vaneechoutte, M, Dijkshoorn, L, Nemec, A, Kämpfer, P, & Wauters, G. Acinetobacter, Chryseobacterium, Moraxella, and Other Nonfermentative Gram-Negative Bacteria. In: Versalovic J, Carroll K, Funke G, Jorgensen JH, Landry ML, Warnock W. Manual of clinical microbiology. 10th ed. Washington, DC: American Society for Microbiology Press, (2011). , 770-779.

[27] Villegas, M. V, & Hartstein, A. I. Acinetobacter outbreaks, 1977-2000. Infect Control Hosp Epidemiol. (2003). , 24, 284-95.

[28] Villegas, M. V, & Hartstein, A. I. Acinetobacter Outbreaks, 1977-2000. Infect Control Hosp Epidemiol. (2003). , 24, 284-295.

[29] Visca, P, Seifert, H, & Towner, K. J. Acinetobacter infection--an emerging threat to human health. IUBMB Life. (2011). Dec;, 63(12), 1048-54.

[30] WHO Guidelines on Hand Hygiene in Health CareGeneva: World Health Organization. (2009).